THE PSORIASIS HANDBOOK

THE PSORIASIS HANDBOOK

A definitive guide to the causes, symptoms and all the latest treatments

Jenny Lewis

with The Psoriasis Association

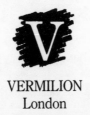

VERMILION
London

Although every effort has been made to ensure that the contents of this book are accurate, it must not be treated as a substitute for qualified medical advice. Always consult a duly qualified medical practitioner. Likewise, you must not regard the suggestions as a substitute for qualified medical advice. Neither the Author, the Publisher nor The Psoriasis Association can be held responsible for any loss or claim arising out of the use, or misuse, of the suggestions made or failure to take medical advice.

First published 1996

1 3 5 7 9 10 8 6 4 2

Copyright © Jenny Lewis 1996

Jenny Lewis has asserted her right to be identified as the author of this work in accordance with the Copyright, Designs and Patents Act 1988.

All rights reserved. No part of this publication may be reproduced, stored in a retrieval system, or transmitted in any form or by any means, electronic, mechanical, photocopying, recording or otherwise, without prior permission of the copyright owner.

First published in the United Kingdom in 1996 by Vermilion
an imprint of Ebury Press
Random House
20 Vauxhall Bridge Road
London SW1V 2SA

Random House Australia (Pty) Limited
20 Alfred Street, Milsons Point, Sydney,
New South Wales 2061, Australia

Random House New Zealand Limited
18 Poland Road, Glenfield,
Auckland 10, New Zealand

Random House South Africa (Pty) Limited
PO BOX 337, Bergvlei, South Africa

Random House UK Limited Reg. No. 954009

A CIP catalogue record for this book is available from the British Library

WW10   ISBN: 0 09 180985 1

Typeset in Monotype Century Old Style
Printed and bound in Great Britain by Mackays of Chatham plc, Kent

Papers used by Ebury Press are natural, recyclable products made from wood grown in sustainable forests.

CONTENTS

FOREWORD

A comprehensive book on psoriasis is long overdue. Now Jenny Lewis has provided us with a far-ranging book, which answers most questions about this most distressing and puzzling condition.

Interviews with those who have coped with the condition are most valuable and eye-opening.

It is important that not only those who suffer from the condition should be well informed, but also anyone who has any dealings with psoriasis sufferers, including health professionals.

This book will also provide a reference point for those studying hairdressing, beauty therapy, alternative therapies, etc., as well as nursing, physiotherapy, occupational therapy, podiatry and so on.

January 1996

LINDA HENLEY
Chief Executive
The Psoriasis Association

INTRODUCTION

Psoriasis is a common skin condition that affects about two percent of the population. Some people will have a mild form of the condition while for others it can be extremely troublesome. As with most chronic illnesses, the severity of psoriasis in any one person can fluctuate enormously.

Although the basic causes of psoriasis are as yet unknown, it is thought that a predisposition to it tends to run in families. It has been estimated that just under a third of sufferers have relatives who also have the condition. If a member of your family has it, you will not necessarily get it. What you have inherited is a susceptibility to it, although doctors do not as yet know exactly why.

Scientists working on identifying the genes that may cause psoriasis currently believe that the condition is not caused by a single gene but by defects in several genes. Environmental factors are also thought to play a part.

*One thing we do know is that psoriasis is **not** caused by poor skin hygiene, nor is it infectious. **You cannot catch it from anyone and, by the same token, no one can catch it from you**.*

Psoriasis is **not** a form of skin cancer. It is an autoimmune disease. This is a condition where the immune system triggers an attack on parts of the body. There are several autoimmune conditions; diabetes is another one.

Psoriasis can develop at any age, with puberty being a common time for it to make its first appearance. It can start in childhood, young adulthood, middle age and even as late as the fifties and sixties, although with people who have a family history of psoriasis, it tends to start at an earlier age. Although throughout the book, psoriasis patients are generally referred to as 'he', this is simply for convenience: psoriasis affects men and women more or less equally. Some women find that it gets better during pregnancy while others find it can occur for the first time in pregnancy. Other women experience psoriasis for the first time during the menopause.

Psoriasis develops when the body produces new skin cells at a much more rapid rate than usual. Normally, the body produces new cells in time to replace the dead ones that have been shed. This is usually a fairly slow and co-ordinated process. With psoriasis, the new skin cells are produced while the dead ones are still on the surface of the skin. The new cells push their way up to the top of the skin forcing the dead cells out. This is what causes the flakiness and gives the psoriatic patches their raised look.

Psoriasis can resemble eczema, a more common skin condition. But the treatment is different. Some of the creams that help eczema do not have any effect on psoriasis and can sometimes even make it worse. The skin condition may be neither psoriasis nor eczema but fungal. Again the treatment is different. So it is very important to get your skin condition expertly diagnosed.

Your GP may be able to diagnose psoriasis by the look of the skin and by finding out whether or not there is a history of psoriasis in your family. If there is any doubt, your doctor will refer you to a dermatologist to confirm the diagnosis.

It is often thought that psoriasis is not an itchy condition, but this is not the case for many sufferers. The Psoriasis Association says that over 50% of patients experience itching and people with scalp psoriasis can be particularly troubled by itchiness. Psoriasis comes from the Greek word 'Psora' which means 'itch'. So itching is an integral part of the condition.

Even though we don't know what actually causes psoriasis, we do have pointers as to some of the things than can set it off for the first time in susceptible people. One of the most common of these seems to be severe emotional stress or trauma. This is discussed further in the next chapter and in different contexts throughout the book. Another possible trigger is a type of throat infection caused by a bacterium called streptococcus which can be followed by a form of the condition known as guttate psoriasis. Most throat infections are viral and not bacterial. Triggers are examined more closely in Chapter One (see pages 13–15).

Although psoriasis cannot be cured, it can be treated and many sufferers find that the condition can go into remission for months and often for years at a time. Some fortunate people find that their psoriasis suddenly goes away and never returns. Getting the condition diagnosed and treated is the key to getting it under control. One of the purposes of this book is to help you to get the better of your psoriasis. Understanding the causes and triggers and knowing how to treat it both with medical help and on your own can help to keep the condition at a containable level.

Since stress and emotions are thought to play such a significant part in psoriasis, this book examines possible treatments in this respect. If, for instance, the condition was initially triggered by a traumatic event, psychotherapy or counselling may be effective ways of treating it. If the psoriatic flare-ups coincide with times of stress or if a stressful life-style keeps the condition constant or severe, finding ways of handling stress is certainly worth a try. All of this is discussed in Chapters Eight and Twelve .

Inevitably, the worst aspect of psoriasis is the psychological effect that it has on sufferers. Many feel that their skin is unsightly and they are embarrassed about it. Some people restrict their social lives considerably because of the embarrassment factor. Many patients will not take part in any activity where communal changing is involved.

One sufferer said she never went swimming. She could ignore the stares at the psoriatic blemishes on her body but she could not cope with the embarrassment in the changing rooms. 'I would take off a vest or a tee shirt and volumes of dead skin would drop,' she explained. 'People would look revolted. Some would quickly leave. It was very hurtful but I couldn't blame them'. Another psoriatic swimmer was asked to leave the swimming pool because her presence was upsetting to the other swimmers.

It is not surprising that many patients feel very isolated despite the fact that in Britain alone there are more than a million people with the condition.

A chronic illness that makes you feel unattractive, uncomfortable and, at times, embarrassed can be very demoralising and this can in itself make the condition worse. But inasmuch as negative feelings can make the psoriasis worse, positive ones can make it better. If you believe that you can get the condition under enough control to live life the way you want to, that is precisely what you will do. It may take time and a lot of trial and error to find the treatments that suit you best, but you will get there and it will be worth the struggle.

This book is written with the co-operation and backing of The Psoriasis Association which represents some 12,000 sufferers in the U.K. Some of the members of the Association have given personal accounts of what it feels like to have psoriasis and how it affects their lives. These stories appear throughout the book.

So, along with medical information, practical advice on how to control the condition and a look at some of the complementary therapies that may help, this book explains what it feels like to have psoriasis. This may enable you to realise that some of the experiences and feelings that you have are shared by a great many others. As you read the personal stories in this book you will probably identify with many of the people who tell them. Often the first bit of healing occurs when you know that you are not alone.

1

WHAT IS PSORIASIS?

Since psoriasis is a condition of the skin and much of what happens is an abnormal functioning of it, let's have a look at this, the largest organ of the body:

· *The Skin* ·

Skin is the largest organ in the body. Its main function is to contain the internal organs and to protect them from the hazards of the outside world. It also keeps the body fluids from oozing out.

Skin consists of two layers: an outer layer called the epidermis and an inner one called the dermis. The epidermis is made up of millions of tiny cells which are constantly being reproduced and this takes place at around the junction of the dermis and the epidermis. As the new cells are formed they push their way up to the top of the skin where they die and form the outer layer which we all see. These dead cells are shed a little at a time.

In normal skin this replenishing of cells takes about 28 days. With psoriasis the new ones push up to the surface of the skin much more quickly, taking about four days. So the epidermis not only houses many more cells but the structure is different. The cells on the skin surface of psoriasis sufferers are newer and they stick together instead of falling off as the older ones do. This increased number of cells in the epidermis is what gives the skin its thick look and these younger stuck together cells make the skin look scaly.

The dermis contains nerve fibres and blood vessels. Nerve fibres produce sensation while the blood vessels do the fetching and carrying of nutrients to the skin. In psoriasis the blood vessels in the dermis are wider than usual and the blood flows much more quickly, increasing the blood supply to the skin. This is what creates the redness in the patches of psoriasis and makes them bleed more easily.

An unusual feature that appears in the dermis of psoriasis sufferers is a larger than normal quantity of white blood cells. Inasmuch as red blood cells have the job of transporting oxygen around the body, white blood cells are the hand-maidens of the immune system. They come into action when the body feels threatened by foreign substances, like, for instance, bacteria or an allergy-producing item. Why white blood cells accumulate in the skin in psoriasis is not known, but it is one reason why some scientists believe that psoriasis may be caused by a particular defect of the immune system.

Sweat glands and sebaceous (oil) glands also appear in the dermis, as do hair follicles. Collagen and other elastic fibres which appear in the dermis give the skin its elasticity and pliability. As we grow older, we have less collagen and elastic fibres in our skin which is why it loses its elasticity and also its resilience.

In the bottom layer of the epidermis are cells known as the Melanocytes. These cells produce skin pigmentation and determine your skin colour and your ability to tan. Again, psoriasis has an effect. If the cells are damaged, the level of pigmentation they produce changes, sometimes producing increased pigmentation which makes the skin look darker, and at other times the condition can cause the Melanocytes temporarily to stop pigment production which has the opposite effect. Both these situations are reversible.

Skin plays an important part in temperature control. If psoriasis is extensive, this function can be impaired and you can find that you fluctuate from feeling too hot to too cold. The skin regulates temperature through blood vessels by increasing or decreasing blood flow. In hot weather when the blood flow method does not cool down the body quickly enough, the sweat glands help out. When this mechanism is not working well enough, as can happen with severe psoriasis, the patient can feel much colder than normal in the extremities (nose, fingers and toes).

Another important point to know is that when psoriasis is severe, there is a rapid flow of blood to the skin to keep it warm. The heat control mechanism, which normally shuts down the blood flow to the skin to keep the centre of the body warm, is not functioning properly. So when you are exposed to the cold you may not feel it as acutely as someone who does not have psoriasis. But what is happening is that your core body temperature is dropping without you being aware of it. This puts you at greater risk of getting hypothermia.

By acting as a barrier, skin protects the internal organs from infection. When psoriasis is severe and the lesions extensive, this function of the skin is also impaired. There is a much greater risk of infection being introduced into the body through the damaged, open skin.

Of course one of the skin's most important functions is to keep the body fluids in. Again, when it is extensively damaged as can occur when psoriasis is particularly severe, the skin loses its ability to perform well. So it lets water out much more quickly than normal which is why you may feel constantly thirsty and your skin excessively dry. Regularly drinking non-alcoholic liquids is a good way to counteract this, as is keeping the skin moisturised. When the skin is very dry it cracks which can be both painful and disabling.

Both the water loss and the temperature control situations are temporary and only occur when the psoriasis is particularly severe and are therefore not commonly experienced.

· *Recognising Psoriasis* ·

The different forms of the condition are explained in Chapter Two (see pages 17–20). The most common one is aptly named common (or chronic) plaque psoriasis. This looks like a raised, red plaque-shaped patch on the surface of the skin. The patches can be small or large, round or oval-shaped and they can appear in clusters, and the affected area, which is scaly and a dull dark red or a brighter colour, looks quite different from the normal skin surrounding it. The patches are rough to the touch and one of the most distressing aspects of the condition for the sufferer is the scaliness. Many people do not like to share communal changing rooms or stay overnight anywhere because of the problem of shedding so much skin. Regular moisturising can reduce scaliness to quite a large extent and this is discussed in Chapter Three.

· *Triggers* ·

One of the most common initial triggers for psoriasis is **emotional trauma**. It could be the death of a loved one, a divorce or a bad accident. Anything that has caused an emotional upheaval can trigger the condition for the first time if you have a predisposition to it. This does not mean you are a nervous type of person.

Any number of chronic complaints including eczema, asthma, migraine, ulcerative colitis and irritable bowel syndrome are linked with stress and emotions along with other factors like, for instance, allergy.

One theory is that you inherit a predisposition to one of these illnesses. You may be cruising along quite happily unaware of your inheritance because you have been symptom-less. Then something very upsetting happens and the condition makes its first appearance. Your body has found a physical outlet for the emotional stress. For your neighbour this outlet may be irritable bowel syndrome because of his family's predisposition, whereas for you this may be psoriasis because of your family's predisposition. And, once triggered, the symptoms recur because the body is now set up to deal with stress in this way. The original trigger may have been a large dose of stress but from now on much smaller amounts can be expressed by the body in this way.

Three things now need to be said. The first is that not everyone agrees with this theory. Second, there are other triggers. Third, it is thought that up to 70% of psoriasis sufferers do not have an obvious family history of the condition. Research is currently taking place on the genetic input in psoriasis.

Physical stress can trigger the condition if you are susceptible to it. Working long and arduous hours without sufficient relaxation can undermine your health and set off psoriasis. If you run your health down you will make yourself vulnerable to all kinds of illnesses, including psoriasis. If you have a chronic condition, one of the most important weapons of defence is to take care of your health. Eat nourishing food, take regular exercise and rest. Keep in condition. If you are physically strong and healthy you will be in a much better position to withstand any unexpected stress, emotional or physical, that may come your way. You will be fighting back.

Some **medicines** can trigger psoriasis or aggravate it. These include beta-blockers which can be prescribed for heart problems, high blood pressure or migraine. Non-steroid anti-inflammatory drugs which are often prescribed for arthritis, and Lithium, which is used to treat mental disorders, are both potential triggers. When you are visiting your doctor about another ailment, it is important to tell him or her that you have psoriasis, even if it is currently dormant, so that he or she can avoid prescribing a drug that may set off the condition. Also, some of the drugs used to treat psoriasis don't mix well with other medicines. If you are taking tablets to treat your psoriasis, always remind the doctor that you are on these so that you are not pre-scribed drugs that will cause problems.

Alcohol tends to make psoriasis worse. This does not mean that you have to abstain completely, but you do have to be more careful with your alcohol intake. If you are on Methotrexate tablets to treat psoriasis you would be well advised to avoid alcohol altogether. Methotrexate can damage the liver as, of course, can alcohol. Taking the two would greatly increase your chances of sustaining liver damage.

Throat infections are another common trigger in someone who is susceptible to psoriasis. This usually precedes guttate psoriasis which is described in Chapter Two (see page 18). A particular type of throat infection caused by the streptococcus bacterium can have this effect, not the more usual viral infection. If diagnosed and treated early, the psoriasis can be cleared quickly and many patients will not experience another attack.

Skin injury can trigger psoriasis or make it occur in an area of the body where it hasn't appeared before. Psoriasis sufferers who work with their hands will often find that the condition appears there and is difficult to clear. Obviously, if you can wear protective clothing (gloves, for instance) this will help. Jobs best avoided by psoriasis sufferers are discussed in Chapter Eleven. If you cut or bruise your skin or scratch or pick at it, psoriasis can be the result. Skin infections or sunburn can trigger the condition or make it worse. Obviously, you cannot go through life fearful of setting off psoriasis with everything you do, but it helps to be forewarned so that you can be a little more careful than you would otherwise need to be.

Smoking lowers the body's natural defences and is, as has been well documented, very bad for your general health. If you are working at keeping your body in good condition to withstand flare-ups of psoriasis, smoking will mitigate against this. However, there is no evidence that giving up smoking will improve most forms of psoriasis, but it has been linked with an increased incidence of palmar plantar (pustular) psoriasis which is a rare form of the condition and is described in Chapter Two (see page 19).

Being **overweight** can make psoriasis worse because it can bring on a form of the condition that appears in the folds of the body. Known as flexural psoriasis, it is rather more moist than scaly and is described more fully in Chapter Two (see page 18).

Currently there is no proven link between psoriasis and what you eat and drink, with the exception of alcohol. Obviously, a well planned and nutritious diet will keep you healthier than junk food. But there are no known food triggers for psoriasis.

This is also the case with pets. Whereas it is known that animal dander can trigger conditions like eczema and asthma, this has not been found to be true of psoriasis.

· *Parts of the Body Affected* ·

Psoriasis can affect different parts of the body including the scalp, face, arms, legs, hands, feet, groin and genitals. Not only are different treatments required depending on the part of the body affected, but the social and psychological implications differ. Psoriasis that appears on the face, for instance, will pose a different set of problems from psoriasis on the scalp or in the groin. Chapter Six deals with how to treat the different areas of the body and, where relevant, discusses the social and psychological implications.

· *Current Research* ·

Current international research indicates that psoriasis could be a malfunction of the immune system. The original pointer to this came about when doctors discovered, quite accidentally, that the immunosuppressive drug Cyclosporin was effective in treating psoriasis. Cyclosporin is described in Chapter Four (see page 48).

Scientists believe that people with psoriasis have some malfunctioning T-cells. The latter are a type of white blood cells that do absolutely nothing until they come across a foreign body such as a virus or a fungus. They then spring into action and secrete chemicals that create a lot of skin cells. The doctors hypothesised that in psoriasis sufferers the T-cells were reacting against something in the psoriatic lesion which was contributing to the disease.

Studying the activated T-cells, the doctors involved noticed that chemicals, called cytokines, that are secreted by these cells appear to make the cells grow too quickly. It seemed possible that it was the T-cell reaction that caused the accelerated production and death of skin cells which produce the psoriatic lesions and scales.

It is hoped that this research will lead to better forms of treatment for psoriasis in the future.

2

DIFFERENT TYPES OF PSORIASIS

There are many types of psoriasis, each of which may need a different type of treatment. It is not unusual for patients to experience more than one form of the condition concurrently. Patients with common or chronic plaque psoriasis may also have some patches of flexural psoriasis, for instance, or they may develop psoriatic arthritis. On the other hand, a youngster may develop guttate psoriasis a few weeks after having a sore throat and then never have another attack of any form of psoriasis ever again. Others may experience several years of remission and then suddenly develop common plaque psoriasis. Over the years patients can move from one type of psoriasis to another.

Knowing which form of psoriasis you have is usually the first step to treating it, so here are some indications that you may find helpful. The most common form of the condition is:

· *Common Plaque Psoriasis* ·

Also known as psoriasis vulgaris, common (or chronic) plaque psoriasis affects over 90% of sufferers. It appears usually on the scalp, lower back, outsides of the elbows and knees and the shoulders. Common plaque psoriasis is very much an adult condition and is seldom seen in children.

Each psoriatic patch looks like a series of little discs or plaques that have superimposed themselves on to the body. This plaque-like shape is peculiar to this form of the condition and is what gives it its name. The plaques are often round or oval in shape or they may not have a distinct shape but they almost always stand out from the surrounding area of the body. The difference between the normal skin and the area affected by psoriasis can be quite marked. Each patch can start as a very small spot and then get bigger over a period of days or weeks. Individual psoriatic patches can spread and join with each other to affect quite a large area of the body. However, there are always psoriasis-free places where the skin looks normal and this serves to emphasise the condition's appearance.

In a typical flare-up the condition can spread quite quickly over a few days or weeks and then stabilise before gradually disappearing. The psoriatic patches become less red and scaly until they reduce in size or disappear completely. But the trouble is that the whole process can start up again quite soon after the previous patches have gone away, which is what makes the condition so frustrating.

The patches are red and rough to the touch and the affected skin incredibly scaly. Scaliness can be kept to a minimum by regularly moisturising the skin with the relevant creams and ointments. And it is important to keep the skin moisturised even when the psoriatic patches seem to have cleared. Often the skin underneath, which you cannot see, has not yet healed and if you don't treat it the scaliness may return quite quickly.

Common plaque psoriasis is not always itchy, nor is it always an uncomfortable condition, but its appearance, along with the shedding of the skin, can cause many sufferers a great deal of emotional discomfort.

This type of psoriasis often affects the scalp as well as the other areas of the body already mentioned. The ways in which psoriasis affects the scalp are discussed in Chapters Three and Six.

· *Guttate Psoriasis* ·

This usually appears suddenly, often following a bacterial throat infection. It is the form of psoriasis most commonly experienced by children and adolescents. The patches appear usually about two to three weeks after the throat infection and spread quite quickly all over the body apart from the palms of the hands and the soles of the feet. Like common plaque psoriasis, the patches are red and scaly and an attack rarely lasts more than a few weeks. Guttate psoriasis is quite easily treated and 50% of sufferers who receive effective treatment never seem to have another attack. With other patients, common plaque psoriasis can ensue.

· *Flexural Psoriasis* ·

This type of psoriasis only appears in certain parts of the body, known as flexures. These are folds or creases in the body and common sites are the armpits, the skin underneath the breasts and the groin. There is very little scaling, although the patches are inflamed and can feel very sore. Appearing as it does in the folds of the skin, it is more moist than other forms of the condition and can be much more uncomfortable physically.

Patients very rarely experience flexural psoriasis on its own. It is more likely to accompany common plaque psoriasis. Psoriasis sufferers in their middle years or old age are more susceptible to this type of psoriasis as are people who are overweight and have more folds of skin.

· *Localised Pustular Psoriasis* ·

Also known as palmar plantar psoriasis or palmoplantar pustulosis, this condition looks very different from common plaque psoriasis and flexural psoriasis and usually only appears on the soles of the feet and the palms of the hands. In place of the inflamed red, scaly patches are a mass of tiny yellow blisters which can be quite painful and look infected even though there is no infection present. Over a period of days the pustules turn a brownish colour and fall off, often only to be quickly replaced. The production of new pustules to replace the ones that have been shed can go on over a period of years.

· *Erythrodermic Psoriasis* ·

A rare condition, erythrodermic psoriasis is one in which the rash is spread over large sections of the body. The skin is very inflamed which affects its ability to function properly. It does not retain fluid as normal which results in the patient feeling constantly thirsty and being dehydrated. It also impairs the skin's performance in maintaining the body's temperature control. So the sufferer may lose heat easily and be more susceptible to hypothermia (see the section on skin in Chapter One, pages 11–13). This is also a more serious form of the condition and one that needs expert medical management. Since so much of the body is involved it is not likely to be treated effectively through creams and ointments and will almost certainly require drug treatment.

· *Generalised Pustular Psoriasis* ·

This is a rare but serious form of psoriasis which can bring similar problems to those produced by erythrodermic psoriasis, as explained above. The pustules are spread over large sections of the body. They erupt and the skin goes red. The condition is accompanied by a high temperature and the patient may also suffer pains in the joints. The patient is likely to be treated in hospital.

Generalised pustular psoriasis can occur as a result of using a lot of strong steroid creams. But please bear in mind that the condition is rare.

· *Psoriatic Arthritis* ·

Some form of inflammation of the joints, or arthritis, has been found to be present in around 10% of psoriasis sufferers. Some psoriasis sufferers have rheumatoid arthritis as well, but there does not seem to be a link between the two. The incidence of rheumatoid arthritis is the same for psoriasis sufferers as it is for the general population. Rheumatoid arthritis affects the middle joints of the fingers as well as the wrists and ankles.

However, there is a specific illness, known as psoriatic arthritis, which appears only in psoriasis patients. Psoriatic arthritis affects between 5% to 10% of psoriasis sufferers. Having widespread psoriasis on the skin does not mean that you will get psoriatic arthritis. Some people with extensive psoriasis on the skin experience the arthritis in a very mild form while others may have the arthritis much more severely than the skin condition. Of course, the majority of psoriasis patients do not experience psoriatic arthritis at all.

Symptoms are very similar to the more usual form of arthritis with the joints becoming swollen, tender and very painful. The most common sites are the finger joints, toe joints, feet, part of the jaw and spine.

It can be very difficult to distinguish between psoriatic arthritis and other forms of arthritis. Some forms of psoriatic arthritis affect one joint and some affect several joints.

Sometimes diagnosis is made through a blood test to identify a particular antibody which would point to the rheumatoid factor. People whose blood test shows the rheumatoid factor are more likely to have rheumatoid arthritis. With psoriatic arthritis the blood test tends to be negative.

An indication that the condition may be psoriatic arthritis is the state of the patient's nails. 'Psoriatic nail disease is present in about 80% of those with psoriatic arthritis in contrast to probably about 30% of those with psoriasis alone,' says rheumatologist Dr. N.J. McHugh, writing in *Psoriasis*, the journal of the Psoriasis Association (1995). 'Therefore in any individual with possible psoriatic arthritis, who has not yet developed psoriasis, examination of the nails may be important'.

Nail psoriasis can sometimes be accompanied by inflammation in the joint of the finger which houses the nail but it is not particularly usual for the skin condition and the arthritis to appear in the same area of the body.

Psoriatic arthritis can come on at any age. It usually precedes the skin condition but occasionally psoriasis can first appear in its arthritic form. Men and women are equally susceptible but more men tend to get arthritis of the spine. Women can contract it after childbirth or during the menopause, which leads doctors to believe that a change in hormones may be involved. Sometimes injury to a joint can trigger a flare-up of psoriatic arthritis in the same way as injury to the skin can trigger the psoriatic rash.

Good skin care is important both for the rash and the arthritis. Moisturising the skin twice a day prevents drying, helps to keep it supple and this in turn makes it easier to keep the joints mobile. You are less likely to be able to exercise your joints if the skin covering them is dry and cracked. Try to avoid injury to the skin through knocking and bruising.

If you have arthritis in the hands, try putting them in warm soapy water every morning and exercising them for a few minutes. Similarly, if other parts of your body are affected, gentle exercise will help with mobility. But it is important not to stress the joint and inflame it further. You have to strike the right balance and this is where physio-therapy comes in. A physiotherapist can give you a set of exercises to do at home which should keep the affected joints as mobile as possible and at the same time build up your muscles which will help to protect the joints.

Some psoriatic arthritis sufferers experience pains in the neck as well as in the back and this, too, can be accompanied by stiffness.

Pain in the joints is often accompanied by stiffness and is usually worse in the morning, getting better during the day as the body warms and loosens up with activity. This is why it is important to keep the affected joints as mobile as possible with controlled and gentle exercise.

As well as physiotherapy, psoriatic arthritis can be treated with drugs and splints to immobilise severely inflamed joints. It is very important to get it correctly diagnosed and treated as, without proper medical help, the condition can deteriorate. But with proper treatment, psoriatic arthritis is unlikely to result in permanent disability.

Drugs used to treat the condition are the non-steroid anti-inflammatory drugs, sulphasalazine, Methotrexate and sometimes gold injections. Drug treatment is discussed in Chapter Four.

There is a pressure group for psoriatic arthritis called The Psoriatic Arthropathy Support Group (see Useful Addresses, pages 153–5). Arthritis Care and the Arthritis and Rheumatism Council for Research (ARC) are two charities that provide a great deal of information on psoriatic arthritis as well as arthritis. Their addresses are included in this book (see page 153). The Psoriasis Association is currently funding research into psoriatic arthritis.

· *Barbara* ·

Barbara has had psoriasis since she was a teenager. She is now 42 years old. Sixteen years ago, after the birth of her second child, she developed psoriatic arthritis. She has had a hip and knee replacement because of it. In the early 1970's Barbara set up the Gateshead branch of the Psoriasis Association which she ran for 14 years. Barbara has three teenage children. Here is her story.

I thought I had a bad case of dandruff and I tried all the different bottles of shampoo you could find. It didn't get me anywhere so I went to the doctor who told me that I had psoriasis. He gave me a prescription for something I had never seen before. It was a smelly coal tar preparation. I thought everybody would steer clear of me. They wouldn't want to know me.

I didn't know what psoriasis was and being a teenager I didn't ask. I thought it was spelt with an 'S' and I had difficulty in looking it up. Years later I read an article in the Observer which said that the 'P' is silent and so are the sufferers. I have found that to be very true. People hide it all the time. You don't realise that one in 50 people have psoriasis. That's two people on a double-decker bus at Christmas time. Somebody I know consoles themselves by the thought that when they get on a full bus they know somebody else on it has psoriasis. It may not be visible but it's there.

But at the time I thought that the prescription the doctor gave me would work and it did – up to a point. I had psoriasis on my elbows as well as my scalp and the ointment for the elbows stained everything.

I wore light colours so that the flakes from my scalp wouldn't show up so much but, of course, school uniforms are dark in colour and there was no way round that. People would come up to me and say: 'What's the matter with you?' It did nothing for my self-confidence. It was the scales that fell from my scalp to my shoulders and sometimes the psoriasis would creep out around the edge of the scalp. It would also occasionally appear on my eyebrows. It was extremely itchy.

I find that if I drink a glass of sherry I itch anywhere and everywhere. I've had to steer clear of alcohol.

It was socially embarrassing at times. When I was a teenager I remember my mother telling me to go to a salon and get my hair cut short as it would be much easier to manage. So I went along. To me my psoriasis wasn't too bad at the time. The hairdresser who washed and cut my hair said to me: 'The next time you come, bring your own towel and your own shampoo and I'm sure your hair is going to fall out'. I walked down the High Street crying my eyes out. I thought I'm not going back there again.

I know that a lot of people with psoriasis find it very difficult to find a sympathetic hairdresser.

My psoriasis gradually got worse. It was bad after the first child but after the second it went mad. When I came home with the baby I didn't feel at all well. My fingers were swollen up like a bunch of bananas. I couldn't bend them properly. I couldn't do up the nappy pins. I was struggling to hold the baby. I couldn't get down on the floor and my back ached all the time. In the mornings my husband had to push me upright in bed and steer my legs over it and push me again to get me in an upright position.

I went to the doctor and said I couldn't cope. Psoriatic arthritis was diagnosed soon after. The arthritis was on my fingers, lower spine, my knees, feet, legs and ankles. All different parts of my body were hurting and I was taking a lot of painkillers.

When the children were little I couldn't get them in and out of the bath and I couldn't manage a bath myself either. So we had the bath removed and installed a shower instead.

I have recently been put on Methotrexate and sulphasalazine as well as an anti-inflammatory medicine. But I'm still aching. I can move around. Sometimes my daughters tell me that I go too fast but sometimes I go too slowly. You find a rhythm of getting around. If you go very slowly it hurts too much.

I tried to type a letter the other day and I ended up with four days of agony while the ends of my fingers ached so much that anything I touched hurt. I typed because my wrists were hurting and I thought I am not going to be able to hold a pen.

I can cook with a bit of help like extra-sharp knives and the right kind of handles, a food processor and things like that. I've got gadgets galore. I have a high stool so I can sit instead of standing. I've got a special seat at a funny angle that lets me sit by the ironing board and iron. I quite enjoy ironing.

I spend my time going to the chiropodist to have my toe nails cut. I have to have it done professionally because my toes are thick and scaly with psoriasis and they are at funny angles because of the arthritis.

It has been very socially restrictive. My husband will ask me in the morning if I fancy going out tonight and I'll say 'yes', but by the evening he'll take one look at me and say: 'you're not up to it'. Months can go by when we haven't been out or done anything specific. I often imagine I can do things that I can't really do. Or if I push myself to do it I'll be ill for the next couple of days.

I have tried alternative therapies, but they are expensive. I find anything that relaxes you is good. In the last three years I have been going to an ecumenical healing centre in Crowhurst for a week every year. I think it helps because it has Christian counsellors you can talk to. It gives me an inner peace and an ability to cope. I think if you feel better in yourself you manage better.

I believe this illness has given me a listening ear to people. I can get along with people who are in a lot of pain which otherwise I may never have done.

I think you have to talk about the illness and how you feel. You can't hide it away or pretend it doesn't exist. For years I used to do that and agree to do things that I couldn't. Now I just say I'm not up to it and I explain why.

An illness like psoriasis and certainly psoriatic arthritis not only affects the patient but all family members. Husbands and wives of sufferers have to cope with extra work in the house as well as social restrictions from time to time. Some may find it hard to be sympathetic with an illness that does not go away completely or, if it does, returns out of the blue. Some may find it hard to be emotionally supportive of their partner when they too are carrying the burden of an illness that is not theirs. Many will find the helplessness of having to stand by while a loved one suffers pain or emotional anguish very difficult to cope with. A problem you cannot solve and a pain you cannot relieve can be tough to live with and very depressing.

Barbara and Tony have been married for 20 years and Tony explains these feelings rather well.

· *Tony* ·

The worst part from a partner's point of view is the knowledge that you can't do anything to relieve the pain or the frustration. Barbara will say 'I wanted to do that with the children', or she would have liked to have gone somewhere or done something and I wouldn't be able to help her do it. And I can't get her over the physical pain.

Very often you can't even give her a cuddle. If her hands are really hurting I can't hold her hand. If her spine is hurting I can't give her a cuddle and say: 'I care'. I just have to put on a cheerful face and that's not always easy.

When the kids were little it was very depressing when Barbara couldn't do up a nappy pin or dress them. Sometimes she couldn't pick the babies or toddlers up. I would worry about what would happen if the kids fell down and I wasn't there. But children are surprisingly resilient and the severity of the condition comes and goes.

When it is bad I am anxious that Barbara will fall down when I'm not there. I worry if she has a knife in her hands that she will cut herself. I'm anxious that she might drop something she is holding and hurt herself and I also worry about the frustration and anxiety she will have if she decides to to something and she fails.

But you've got to make the best of it and put yourself into other things. I read books and go for walks and if I do get depressed, which is inevitable, I go and find a friend to call on and have a drink or a cup of tea and a chat. You've got to have someone to talk to.

It's not always easy to talk to the person who has the illness because they think you are blaming them and maybe you are, partly. And that makes you feel guilty. But if you can talk about your anxieties and frustrations as well as other things it keeps you going.

We've talked more and more about our anxieties. As time has gone on we've realised that the problem is not just the physical pain and the inability to do physical things but a large part is the mental frustration. Talking about it is important.

It is isolating for both of us. The physical problem is there in all dimensions. There are times when you can hold hands and cuddle, but there are times when you can't. You have to make the most of the good times and appreciate them.

There are a lot of places we can't go to. We never go to a dance, because Barbara can't dance. I like dancing and it is an option denied.

We've had to find relaxing things to share. We listen to music, watch TV and listen to radio programmes together. I try to take Barbara out to the cinema or theatre and that can be frustrating because I have to be aware that it may not happen if she is unwell. We can't plan any outing. We have to do it on the spur of the moment.

We enjoy going out together. We live six or seven miles away from a beach. We drive down to the beach, buy an ice cream and walk along. When I say a walk I'm talking tongue in cheek. We walk 150 yards there and 150 yards back.

We have a nice park nearby. We might go there for a walk but the *walks have got to be from seat to seat. It's not a walk that other people might think about. You have to limit your horizons and enjoy what is in that horizon. You learn to appreciate the 150 yards as opposed to the mile and a half.*

Now when I look back I remember that I was annoyed that Barbara couldn't do up the nappy pins, bath the baby or dress the children so I had to do it. It was extremely tiring and annoying. But now I look upon it as a blessing in a sense. I picked my children up and washed them and played games with them more than the average father does and more than I would have planned. I think that has made me much closer to my daughters.

3

TOPICAL TREATMENTS

Treatments for psoriasis include *topical* treatments – ointments and creams that you put directly on to the skin – and *systemic* treatments – tablets or liquids that you take orally. Light therapy can also be used to treat psoriasis.

This chapter discusses topical treatments together with any side effects. Systemic treatments and ultra-violet therapy are discussed in Chapters Four and Five.

Topical treatment is by far the most widely used. Systemic treatment is reserved for the times when the condition is severe and is not being controlled in any other way.

· *Drug Naming* ·

Drugs in general use are known by three different names. The first one is given by the Nomenclature Committee of the British Pharmacopeia Commission which consists of doctors, pharmacologists, pharmacists and chemists. This is the official medical name and it is a generic term for the basic active substance of the drug. The second name is given by the manufacturer.

Different manufacturers will give different brand names to a drug which has the same basic active substance. This is to put their name on it, so to speak. Sometimes the brand name is easier to remember.

Sometimes the basic substance of a drug is combined with other substances to produce a different medication. These drugs are known as compound preparations. Betnovate and coal tar are often combined to provide a compound topical preparation for psoriasis.

The third name is the chemical and technical one. To anyone outside the medical profession it is an incomprehensible mixture of numbers and letters and it need not concern us here.

· *Effect of Moisturisers* ·

Fortunately, many of the creams and ointments that you rub into your skin to treat psoriasis are simple, natural preparations that can be bought over the counter and are used by anyone with dry skin. These are known as *emollients* and are mixtures of water, waxes, fats and oils in varying proportions. They are moisturisers. When the surface of the skin is damaged, it lets the moisture out. The result is dry skin with an increased tendency to crack. Those with psoriasis can also suffer from itchiness.

Applied regularly, moisturisers can provide a film of oil on the skin which helps to prevent the loss of moisture. This film can also act as a barrier against outside irritants and infections. Moisturising the skin makes it soft and gets rid of the scaling. It also makes it less itchy. This is why moisturising is such an important first-line treatment for psoriasis. If you moisturise your skin twice a day you can stop the flaking.

Moisturisers can come in the shape of ointments which are greasy or creams which are not. You can usually choose which you prefer. If the psoriasis patches are very dry, it may be better to go for the ointment, although to avoid greasy patches on your clothes, it may be better to use an ointment at night when it doesn't matter so much and a cream during the day.

Emollients or special oily soaps can also be used in place of ordinary soaps that dry the skin.

Vaseline or petroleum jelly is one of the emollients most commonly used by psoriasis sufferers, as is E45. Baby oil is another simple product that is widely used along with emulsifiers and aqueous creams. However, the ingredient lanolin is not always well tolerated.

Simple emollients used in dermatology do not contain perfume. Moisturisers that contain perfume are a cosmetic rather than a dermatological item. It is possible that the perfume added to a moisturiser may irritate your psoriasis.

If you find that a product you are using inflames your skin, **stop using it**. Find out the ingredients of the particular moisturiser you have been using. This usually appears on the packaging. Look for a moisturiser with different ingredients. Your pharmacist should be able to advise on a suitable emollient for you. Make a note of any moisturisers you have used that have caused problems so that you never use them again.

· *How to Use Moisturisers* ·

Here are some tips on moisturising your skin.

- Moisturise your skin every day, usually at least twice. Sometimes the doctor may suggest that you use the emollients more frequently than that to get the condition under control. Remember that you don't have to moisturise your entire body all the time, just the psoriatic patches.
- A good time to moisturise the skin is just after you've had a bath or shower when the skin is soft and warm. Some people find using a bath oil helpful. This, of course, moisturises the whole body which cannot do you any harm. But be careful not to slip in the bath. *Always make sure that the bath water is warm, not hot.* Also, don't spend too long in the bath as this can dry the skin. Do not scrub the areas of your body affected by psoriasis.
- If you are in a hurry you may find this a quick way of moisturising: stand in the bath while the water is running out and apply some baby oil all over your skin. If you have something else to do before you dry yourself, like, for instance brushing your teeth, wrap a towel around you, brush your teeth, and then gently pat yourself dry. The few minutes you have taken to brush your teeth allows time for the oil to be absorbed into your skin, but if you haven't time for that, it doesn't matter.
- Another good time to apply moisturisers is before you go to bed. This allows plenty of time for the emollient to be absorbed.
- Make sure you are using the right emollient! If you have psoriasis on your scalp as well as elsewhere on your body, the chances are that the doctor will have prescribed two different treatments, one for the body and one for the scalp. To make sure you don't confuse them, label them clearly.
- Always wash your hands before applying the moisturisers and ensure that the lids and tops are firmly closed after use. Psoriatic patches can become infected if the contents of the container are contaminated. You may find a pump dispenser useful.
- Use the creams sparingly. Apply thinly and gently smooth in. If you have several patches to moisturise and the emollient you are using is a thick one, you may find it helpful to apply it in small dots on the affected parts of the body and gently smooth it in patch by patch. By the time you have come to working in the later patches, you should find that the emollient has melted and is easier to use.

- Never rub psoriatic patches or apply the creams harshly.
- Don't be tempted to rub the scales from the patches before moisturising. This is likely to inflame the skin and aggravate the condition. Just gently apply the moisturiser on top of the scales.
- Have a good look at the labels. Follow any usage instructions carefully and check the sell-by date. Any cream or ointment that is older than the date printed on it will have started to lose its efficacy.
- Although ointments and creams can be messy, don't let this put you off using them. Take precautionary measures. Using just a thin film of the product should cut down on excess grease, and if you are applying moisturiser before you go to bed, wear nightwear that you are not worried about spoiling and use old sheets.

    If you are applying moisturiser to your scalp, put a towel on top of the pillow. During the day it is a little more difficult to control. Try to moisturise after a bath, when the cream or ointment will be absorbed faster. Also, if you can wait a few minutes with a towel or bathrobe around you, very little moisturiser will be left to come off on your clothes.
- If you enjoy swimming but it dries your skin, you might find that putting emollient on the patches before you swim helps to counteract dryness. Always shower after you have come out of the water and re-apply the moisturiser.
- Remember, moisturisers do not clear the psoriatic patches but, by keeping them supple, you can cut down on the scaling and can help to reduce the cracking, both of which can make the condition so much worse.
- Don't expect immediate results. It takes a few weeks for the moisturisers to work so you will need to persevere.

    Keep moisturising the skin even if the patches seem to have cleared. It may not have healed underneath the skin surface. If you run your fingers over the skin you may be able to feel the edges of the plaques even though the skin looks clear. You need to carry on moisturising at least until the skin feels completely smooth.

    Carry on moisturising your skin on a daily basis even when the psoriasis is clear. Keeping your skin moist, soft and supple not only helps it to look nice, but prevents it from becoming dry and more open to injury.

    Some simple moisturisers that have been found to be useful by members of The Psoriasis Association are: Neutrogena, Vaseline intensive care, Aloe Vera and E45, but there are many others.

· *Salicylic Acid* ·

Salicylic acid works by removing the layers of dead skin cells. It is particularly useful for treating crusts and thick scale in scalp psoriasis. It is often used as a compound preparation, i.e., mixed with another active ingredient in a cream or ointment to produce a more dramatic effect. In hospitals, many of the preparations used to treat psoriasis have salicylic acid in their formulations.

· *Tar* ·

Sometimes emollients are mixed with active ingredients to bring about more positive results. These are used to clear up the psoriatic patches and should only be used on the psoriatic patches. (You should wash your hands before and after using these preparations.)

The oldest emollient is the one containing tar and it is still widely and effectively used for psoriasis.

Tar is made by distilling wood or coal to produce a strong-smelling thick black liquid. A small quantity of this concentrated liquid is mixed into an emollient to produce a preparation that you can use on your skin. An alternative is coal tar solution, where the water soluble chemicals are extracted from the tar. Coal-tar solutions are not as messy as concentrated tar ones but are not quite as effective either.

Tar-based preparations to treat psoriasis include creams, ointments, gels, bath additives as well as shampoos and lotions to treat psoriasis of the scalp. (More on treating scalp psoriasis in Chapter Six, pages 61–4.)

Tar-based preparations you may have heard of include Polytar, Clinitar and Alphosyl. Some preparations combine tar with another active ingredient to produce an add-on effect. For instance, tar can be combined with salicylic acid which helps to reduce the scale. Psorin is one of these.

Although modern tar treatments are much more user-friendly than the older crude coal-tar preparations, they can still be a little smelly and troublesome to use. But they seldom cause any side effects. However, if you are prescribed a tar preparation and you find it does inflame or irritate your skin, stop using it and go back to the doctor.

Let's assume that you have been prescribed a tar preparation that is smelly, messy to use and could stain your clothing. However, there is a very good chance that the tar is going to heal your psoriasis, so how do you minimise the problems?

Applying the ointment before you go to bed is one good step. If the affected area of your body is somewhere that you can bandage, try that. It should save your bedclothes. You can buy tubular bandages from chemists that are much more effective than the wind-around bandages. They are easier to put on, and since they won't unravel, they are more likely to stay in place. But you should be careful not to buy a bandage that is tight. This will only make your skin itchy and sore. Failing that, use old bed-clothes. Remember you won't be doing this for ever and the results could be very worthwhile.

If you need to apply the tar solution during the day as well as at night, try the bandaging method or, again, wear old cotton, loose-fitting clothing next to your skin.

This form of tar treatment which you apply yourself at home can take between a month to six weeks to work. And it is a gradual process. You should notice a slight general improvement in your skin. Eventually, the psoriatic patches should clear completely, leaving a slight reddishness where they once were for a few weeks afterwards.

Some points you need to bear in mind when using tar preparations at home:

• Only use them on the areas of your body affected with psoriasis.
• Keep the preparation away from your eyes.
• Wash your hands before and immediately after use.

Don't be tempted to keep old jars of preparation after you have finished with them. It may be tempting to store them in case the psoriasis comes back so that you can treat it straight away. But the preparation will lose its potency with age, so it's better to get a new one. And can you be sure that the current skin problem is psoriasis again? It's better to go back to your doctor and get the right treatment. It should save you a lot of trouble in the long run.

A tar treatment that speeds up the process already described is the **Goeckermann regimen**, named after the American doctor who invented it. It is very rarely used in this country, but basically what happens is that tar ointments and baths with tar solution are used in combination with ultra-violet light (see Chapter Five, pages 54–6). The ointment has to be removed before you go under the ultra-violet light. The Goeckermann treatment is usually carried out daily for two to three weeks.

· *Dithranol* ·

Dithranol is a man-made chemical and one of the most effective treatments for psoriasis, but it does have its drawbacks: it can burn the skin and it can stain clothing indelibly. However, since it can work particularly well to treat common plaque psoriasis, it is definitely worth considering. So let's take a closer look at it.

Dithranol is thought to reduce the excessive production of new skin cells which causes the psoriatic scaliness. It used to be administered mainly in hospitals but now with the improvement in the creams it can be used at home.

The amount of dithranol included in the emollient differs from person to person. Some people can tolerate less than one percent of active ingredient in the preparation while others can take up to 10 percent.

There are three methods of treatment using dithranol.

The first is known as **short contact therapy** and can be used at home. The ointment or cream comes in different strengths and often the prescription your doctor gives you will include two preparations of different strengths. (You will pay only one prescription charge for this.)

This preparation is applied once a day to the psoriatic patches and is left on for 30 minutes. You need to be careful not to get the ointment on the surrounding unaffected skin because it can irritate or burn it. Protect the surrounding areas with a thick layer of simple emollient. Vaseline works well.

Gently rub a small amount of the cream into each psoriatic patch until it has been absorbed. (You may want to wear thin, well-fitting polythene gloves to prevent the dithranol getting on to your fingers.) When the 30 minutes are up, wash the cream off.

If you are using the dithranol for your scalp, you should first comb your hair to remove the loose scales. Then part the hair in the appropriate places and rub the preparation into the psoriatic areas. After 30 minutes, shampoo it off. People with fair hair may find that it takes on a pinkish tinge. This will grow out when you stop the treatment.

Dithranol can also stain the skin, turning it a purple-brown. Please do not be tempted to scrub the staining from your skin. It will fade gradually after you have finished the treatment.

If you want to get the staining off towels and dressing gowns, you can try using soda crystals. Soak them in water to which you have added soda crystals or just put the crystals in the washing machine.

Dithranol burning is similar to sunburn in how it looks and feels. Burning is prevented by using the same principles as you would to prevent sunburn. You have to get your skin used to the chemical by starting with a preparation with a very small amount of active ingredient and then gradually increasing it as your skin becomes more resistant. As with sunburn, people with fair skin, blond or red hair are more susceptible to burning.

Should you experience burning or soreness at any stage, you will need to reassess the treatment. Depending on the severity of the burning, you may need to treat the condition with just moisturiser until the soreness subsides or cut back to a lower strength preparation. Needless to say, you should seek your doctor's advice at this stage.

Dithranol is not suitable for use on the folds or creases in the skin: under the breasts, in the neck, groin or armpits, or the genital area where it is more likely to burn. Although it can be used on the face, most patients avoid it because of the staining.

The treatment usually takes between four to six weeks to clear the psoriasis, but it varies from person to person.

It is particularly important to throw away any unused containers of dithranol preparation once you have completed the treatment. It is not a stable substance and goes off quite quickly, so if the colour of the preparation has gone a purple-brown, throw it away. Also, it is essential to get the treatment prescribed afresh using the quantity of active ingredient that the doctor thinks fits the current state of your psoriasis. Never use other people's treatments. They may be too strong for you and inflame your skin badly.

Dithrocream and Alphodith are two brand names of short contact dithranol treatments.

The second form of treatment is one that is used in hospital. The active ingredient is mixed with a thick paste and applied to the patches. Patients often wear light bandages which helps to maximise the effect of the preparation. This is often left on for several hours every day over a period of two or three weeks.

Pioneered by British dermatologist John Ingram, the third form of treatment is called the **Ingram regimen**. This treatment uses dithranol preparations accompanied by ultra-violet therapy. The dithranol boosts the effect of ultra-violet therapy. This treatment is given in hospital either on an in-patient or a day-care basis.

· *Cortisone Creams* ·

Cortisone is a corticosteroid and steroids are a group of natural hormones produced by the body. They reduce inflammation and itching and help the healing process by suppressing the symptoms. Artificially produced steroids aim to have the same effect. They are now widely available in creams and ointments and can be used to treat psoriasis.

(Incidentally, corticosteroids are quite different from the anabolic steroids used by some athletes and body builders.)

The advantage of topical (i.e. applied externally) steroids is that they are easy to use. There is no mess or staining. The disadvantage is that once you stop the treatment, the psoriasis usually comes back quite quickly and sometimes worse than it was before. If you use steroids continually for several months your psoriasis can become resistant to the strength of the active ingredient in the preparation. So you will have to increase the potency. It is thought that excessive use of steroids over a number of years can, in some cases, result in common plaque psoriasis becoming generalised pustular psoriasis which, as we discussed in the previous chapter, is a much more severe condition.

However, having said that, there is a place for topical steroids in the treatment of psoriasis. The unwanted side effects commonly associated with steroids occur when this treatment is taken internally, either in tablet form or by injection which is very rarely prescribed for psoriasis. The side effects of systemic (i.e. taken orally) steroids are mentioned on pages 44–51.

Topical steroids are useful for treating psoriasis on the folds of the skin as in flexural psoriasis. If you have patches of psoriasis on your face you can consider using a **mild** steroid cream to clear those up. However, you should not use steroid creams on your face without medical supervision and definitely not for any length of time. As a short-term treatment it could be helpful.

Short-term treatment with steroid creams may also be helpful for treating psoriasis in the genital area and on the scalp.

In summary, corticosteroids can be helpful in treating psoriasis providing they are used with a certain amount of care. The problem is that once treatment stops the condition often returns and it can be tempting to resume applying the creams and ointments. It is this cycle that you need to be careful to avoid. Not only are the steroids not curing the psoriasis but the latter may be becoming resistant to the treatment.

Don't keep old tubes of treatment. Throw them away once you have finished with them. It is better to go back to the doctor and see whether or not he or she is prepared to prescribe this form of treatment again.

Here is a general guide to the potency levels of different topical steroids. *Please note that by no means all the preparations available are listed here and this is just intended as an indication.*

Very Potent

The following creams are generally not suitable for young children and older children should only use them for short periods of time. They should not be used on the face or eyelids or without medical advice. Apply a very thin smear with one fingertip to the affected area once or twice a day at the most. If you are using this strength you should keep in regular contact with your doctor.

Dermovate	Halciderm
Dermovate NN	Nerisone Forte

Potent

The same comments apply for this potency as for very potent.

Adcortyl	Nerisone
Betnovate	Propaderm
Diprosone	Synalar
Elocon	Topilar
Locoid	

Moderately Potent

These can be used for longer periods and very occasionally on the face. They can be used for a short time on young children when the psoriasis is severe. Use sparingly on the psoriatic patches only, once or twice a day and keep in touch with your doctor.

Alphaderm	Haelan
Betnovate RD	Stiedex LP
Calmudrid HC	Synalar 1:4
Eumovate	

Mildly Potent

These are generally safe, but should only be used for very short periods on the very young.

Canesten HC

Efcortelan

Epifoam

Fucidin H

Gentisone HC

Hydrocortistab

Hydrocortisyl

Mildison Lipocream

Quinocort

Synalar 1:10

Tarcotin

Terra-cortril

Terra-Cortril nystatin

Timodine

Guidelines for the use of topical steroids for psoriasis appeared in the *British Medical Journal* on 5 October 1991 (volume 303). The recommendations were:

● There should be regular clinical review.
● No unsupervised repeat prescriptions should be made.
● No more than 100g of a British National Formulary Grade III (moderately potent) preparation should be applied each month.
● There should be periods each year when alternative treatment is employed.
● Use of British National Formulary grade I (very potent) or grade II (potent) preparations should be under dermatological supervision.

· *Calcipotriol* ·

This is a relatively new topical treatment specifically developed for moderate to mild psoriasis, and is sold under the brand name of Dovonex. It is available as an ointment, cream and scalp solution.

A derivative of vitamin D, Calcipotriol is particularly effective for common plaque psoriasis. Vitamin D helps to regulate the level of calcium and phosphate in the body. It is, of course, essential for maintaining strong bones and teeth.

Calcipotriol is thought to work by reducing the excessive reproduction of skin cells that causes the thickening and scaling and produces the psoriatic patches. It has a very real advantage over dithranol and coal tar in that it doesn't stain or smell. But calcipotriol can irritate the skin and produce a rash on the face even if it is not being applied there. If you experience a rash on a part of your body that is not being treated with calcipotriol, you should contact your doctor.

You need to be careful to apply the preparation only to the affected areas of the body. So be sure to wash your hands thoroughly after using the ointment.

An excessive use of calcipotriol can raise the level of calcium in your body which can cause problems. This can happen if the psoriasis is widespread and therefore the amount of active ingredient being absorbed into the body is relatively high for a topical treatment. However, if you are using quantities of less than 100 grams of topical calcipotriol per week, which is the maximum recommended (most patients need considerably less than 20 grams per week), you should not experience any problems.

· *Tacalcitol* ·

This new treatment is marketed under the brand name of Curatoderm and, like calcipotriol, is a vitamin D derivative. It works by slowing down new cell production. Tacalcitol needs only to be applied once every 24 hours and it should be used sparingly. Apply it thinly to the affected areas only. One fingertip unit is enough ointment to cover one hand. Two-and-a-half fingertip units will cover the face and neck. (A fingertip unit is the amount of ointment it takes to cover an adult finger from its tip to the crease of the next joint.)
Tacalcitol is best used at night as exposure to sunlight may make it less effective. It can be used on the face. Although the time it takes to work varies from patient to patient, an improvement in the look and feel of the skin may be experienced in about two weeks.

· *Mary* ·

Mary comes from a line of psoriasis sufferers. Her mother has it, but quite mildly, and she believes that her great grandmother had it too. Mary has used dithranol in the past in hospital and at home. She has two daughters aged ten and eight. Here is her story.

When I was 16 I had a major row with my mother and psoriasis came out on my elbows and my knees. It's common plaque psoriasis.

I have had it ever since. During both my pregnancies it disappeared only to come back after each baby was born. Four months after the birth of my younger daughter it came back in the state it is now. And it is quite bad.

I have psoriasis from my knees down and it's even on the front of my feet. It's the same with my arms. It's there from my elbows down to the front of my hands. It's one mass of red. But it is not on my body or my face and I very rarely get it in my hair.

I don't let it bother me. I'm lucky. I don't need to wear posh things for work. I am the manager of a fireplace showroom. It's quite a dirty job so I can wear jeans. I always wear long-sleeved blouses. At work I am okay. Nobody notices but I do get comments from time to time about the bits on my hands.

It really gets to me in summer because I still have to cover up then and that bugs me. And when I go out in the evening I see everybody wearing slinky things and there's me in my same black cocktail pants.

My psoriasis is not itchy. I think that's because I loofah it in the bath. I think with the plaque type of psoriasis it is the scales getting caught in your clothes that make you itch. It makes you pick at it. I don't go mad, but I put some emulsifier on a loofah and I rub it gently. When I get out of the water I always slap some cream on my hands and moisturise the areas with psoriasis. I do that every day. I try my best to keep it flat at all times and I moisturise so that the scales don't appear. I very rarely get scales. It means that I'm not walking around dropping bits of skin every-where.

I had a course of UVB in the hospital which worked in conjunction with dithranol. I was in hospital for three weeks. You all stand there and paint each other's spots with dithranol. It's so boring being in hospital that you want to make yourself useful so you put the treatment on one another. It's much quicker and it's quite funny really.

I had to put tubigauze over my arms and legs. In those days you had to keep it on for eight hours. You wandered around with that stuff on for that time and then you showered. And the next day you did the whole thing all over again. I don't think you have to keep the dithranol on for so long these days. During the last week I had the UVB treatment. And after I was discharged I went back as an out-patient for UVB every other day for a month. And that was that.

I was totally clear when I left the hospital. I went and had a sauna and a Jacuzzi. But I wouldn't do it again. I just can't take three weeks out of my life like that.

I have used dithranol at home since and it is a messy thing to use. It worked but I would get cheesed off with doing it. I'd say goodbye to my husband while he was watching TV. I'd go upstairs, have a shower or bath and put the dithranol on. I'd wear a special pair of pyjamas and just sit there in my bedroom for half an hour and then get back in the shower. It was such a pain. This was the short contact treatment. If I continued to do it I think I would be clear but it takes a long time.

One time we were going to a wedding and I had quite a lot of notice and there was a dress I particularly wanted to wear. So I did the dithranol treatment at home. It took me eight weeks to clear the psoriasis as well as the little black marks that the dithranol left behind. But I did wear the dress and it was fine but within months the psoriasis was back again.

I am very fair-skinned. I have to be careful in the sun because I burn but, to be honest, I don't want to take my clothes off in the first place. My mother tells me I should go swimming or go on to the beach wearing a bikini because no one will look, but they do. She has psoriasis but only in little patches and it's not the same.

I came to the conclusion about 15 years ago that the people who matter to me and know me accept me as I am. They know what I've got and we don't even talk about it. They're the only people worth knowing anyway.

Luckily for me my husband is very good. He knew me before I had the psoriasis so he's lived with it getting worse and worse. It doesn't bother him at all. It bothers me more than it bothers him.

I used not to explain to people what it was. I would say I'd burnt myself and they'd accept that right away. It's mind boggling. I'd say it's eczema. People know what eczema is and so they accept it. But once you start saying it's psoriasis they say 'what's that?' They don't know what it is and they think you're leperish. You try to tell them it's not contagious but they're already shuffling away.

My life's ambition at the moment is to take my children swimming before they hit their twenties. I want to actually get in the water with them. I've never done that. I've always had to sit and watch. But some time in the next 10 years I am going to swim with them.

· *Dave* ·

Dave is 51 years old and has had psoriasis for 30 years. He first experienced it when he was in the Forces and was working in South America. It appeared on his scalp in a mild form. It has been considerably worse since then. Dave is very involved with the Southampton branch of the Psoriasis Association which he helped to start 12 years ago. He is married and has a nine-year-old daughter. Here is his story.

My psoriasis got much worse in the early 1970s after my mother died. I think it was the shock. What happened was that I had served nine years in the army pay Corp. and when I came out I went to work in Saudi Arabia for a while. The job wasn't what I had expected it to be and I resigned after about five months and came back to England. I wasn't married then and so I came home to my parents' house. When I knocked on the door there was no answer and a neighbour told me that my mother was in hospital and my father was there with her.

I went to the hospital and saw that my mother was in a bad way. She died a few days later. It was a big shock because I had no forewarning. My father had written to me to say that my mother had been taken ill but the letter had crossed with me coming home. It was coincidental really. The letter eventually caught up with me back in England but by that time my mother was dead.

After that my psoriasis got progressively worse and over the years it has been pretty bad. At one stage I had it very badly in the scalp. The psoriasis was on the hairline at the front and it was visible if I combed my hair back. It looked like very bad dandruff and showed up on the shoulders if I wore a dark suit. When I combed my hair I'd find a lot of scaly stuff on my clothes.

I got married for the first time in 1973 and I went through a period when I had to massage a horrible coconut oily substance into my scalp at night time and wear a shower cap because it was so messy. I had to put special pillow cases on because some of it used to come through. Every day I had to take it off again before I went to work.

My wife was very supportive. She used to help me with the creams on my back. But it embarrassed me. It was probably a bit of a masculine thing really and there was a big age difference between us. I was 30 and my wife was 20 and I suppose I felt embarrassed about having to admit to a deficiency. She was very good about it. But men don't like to admit to failings in themselves. Looking back with hindsight you see things differently.

They took me into hospital for a week to try and sort it out. They put on some sort of cream that burned. It was something that at the time they didn't like you to apply yourself. Every night the nurse used to come around and put the stuff on to my scalp and I'd have to shampoo it off the next morning. I don't think it has ever come back as badly as that again.

Psoriasis has never really left me since the early 1970s. The psoriatic arthritis started then as well. That was a bit of a blow because when I was in the army I was quite active. I used play football and do cross-country running. Suddenly in my early thirties I realised that my knees were getting stiff. My knees were never a site for the rash.

My doctor told me that I wasn't going to end up in a wheelchair. He assured me that I was not going to be crippled which was what I was worried about.

I still have the psoriatic arthritis and it affects the elbows, knees and soles of the feet. It tends to stiffen up at night. When I have a particularly bad patch of it, it takes me a little while to get going in the mornings. At the moment I am having trouble with my wrists. They have stiffened up quite a lot and they can be quite painful. But with the arthritis, as with the rash, you go through good and bad times. It can be very painful for a while and then it subsides. In the summer during the very hot spell that we had I went through a very bad patch for a couple of weeks. I find that the heat makes it worse.

The arthritis is the worst part for me. The rash I can cover up. Unless I tell someone I have psoriasis they wouldn't know. But when I am going through a bad patch with the arthritis it restricts my mobility. Since it is on the soles of my feet and my knees it can be painful to walk. But generally it doesn't stop me doing anything. You tend to adapt to a situation. Perhaps I lift things in a different way. I still do the decorating and the gardening. But I don't do sport any more.

The rheumatologist I see is very good. He takes a great interest and explains things. That along with getting involved with the Psoriasis Association helps a lot. It's good therapy talking to people with the same illness and being able to help some of them sometimes. Also it takes a lot of the fear out of an illness when you understand what it is.

4

TAKING THE TABLETS

Doctors prefer to treat a condition like psoriasis with topical medicine. Creams and ointments that you put on your skin are less likely to enter the bloodstream than drugs that you swallow. And even if they do get absorbed internally they are bound to do so in smaller quantities. But when the psoriasis is severe and is not responding well enough to topical treatment, or is on a part of the body that is difficult to treat topically, oral medicines may be used. Psoriasis on the hands or genital area are two examples. Or it may be that psoriasis covers such a large part of your body that creams and ointments are not a practical option.

Many of the systemic drugs used to treat psoriasis have side effects and some of these can be serious ones if the medicine is taken in sufficient quantities over a period of time. So doctors are generally reluctant to prescribe them unless the severity of the condition warrants it. It is very important to know as much as you can about the drug you have been prescribed.

Most of the drugs used for psoriasis are ones that have been developed for treating other conditions. For instance, both Methotrexate and Hydroxyurea are anti-cancer drugs that are also used for psoriasis. Both work for psoriasis by slowing down the production of new cells.

Most medicines taken orally get into the bloodstream via the wall of the small intestine. The drug is then transported by blood vessels to the liver where it is turned into a substance that can be used by the body. This substance is now in general circulation in the body. So whereas topical medicines treat only the place or places where the problem occurs, systemic medicines treat the specific trouble spots in the body by absorbing the drug into the whole system. It may seem like using a hammer to crack a nut but sometimes there is no option.

Obviously no one wants to take systemic medicine for any longer than necessary. Following the doctor's instructions is one way to achieve this. Patients sometimes feel that if they do not complete the course of treatment they will be taking less harmful stuff into their system. This may well be so but they may also be delaying the process of recovery and prolonging the treatment.

So rule number one is to take your medicine exactly as prescribed by your doctor. Make sure you know what dose to take and how often you should take it. Should the medicine be taken before or after meals? Drugs taken on an empty stomach are absorbed more quickly into the bloodstream. This may be a good thing for some medicines. However, drugs that are likely to irritate the stomach are better taken after meals to avoid that possibility. Check it out with your doctor.

Some people swallow tablets without fluid. This is very bad practice. Tablets taken without water can get stuck in the oesophagus and not only does this delay the action of the medicine but it can also damage the oesophagus. Do not swallow tablets while you're lying down, either. These medicines are best taken standing or sitting up.

Here are some general do's and don'ts when taking oral medicines.

- Find out if you need to complete the prescribed treatment and if so, do it. Otherwise the condition may return and be more difficult to treat.
- Tell your doctor about any drugs that you are already taking. Medicines sometimes don't mix.
- If you experience adverse reactions like nausea, sickness diarrhoea or skin reaction that may have been caused by the medicine prescribed, contact your doctor.
- Some medicines do not mix with alcohol. (Methotrexate described on pages 45–6 is one.) Find out from your doctor if this is the case with the drug you have been prescribed.
- If you are pregnant, thinking of becoming pregnant or at all likely to become pregnant, tell your doctor. Many drugs cannot and must not be taken during pregnancy for fear of harming the baby.
- If you suffer from any other illness apart from psoriasis, you need to tell your doctor. Liver or kidney disease, heart problems, asthma or other complaints may well have a bearing on whether or not a particular drug can be prescribed.
- If you have experienced allergic reactions to any medicine, mention it to your GP.
- Don't take medicines that have not been prescribed for you.
- Make sure all drugs in your household are stored safely out of reach of young children.
- Store drugs in a cool, dry place, preferably away from light and check whether or not they need to be refrigerated.
- Keep all medicines in their original containers and ensure that the drug names and instructions are legible. Confusion, if not disaster,

can arise when you start moving drugs around from container to container.

- Don't keep left-over prescribed tablets to take as and when the condition recurs. Get your doctor's opinion first.
- Don't keep any tablets, even over-the-counter ones, for more than two years.

The following are some of the most commonly used tablets to treat psoriasis. Please remember that these systemic drugs are only used when the condition is severe or not responding to topical treatment.

· *Methotrexate* ·

This is a drug that is normally used for treating certain types of cancer but it is also very effective in treating psoriasis. It has been used to treat psoriasis for more than 40 years. It is also sometimes used for treating psoriatic arthritis. It works for cancer by reducing the speed at which the cells in the body divide and multiply. It works for psoriasis by slowing down the rate at which the new cells are being formed on the skin's surface to produce and maintain the psoriatic patches.

The doses prescribed for psoriasis are very much lower than for cancer. Methotrexate is usually given as a single weekly dose which reduces the side effects.

Methotrexate can damage the liver. People have taken this medicine for years without experiencing this effect but it can happen and it is linked with the state of your liver in the first place and, of course, how much of the drug you have been taking. Short, low-dose treatments do not seem adversely to affect people with healthy livers. Taken over several years Methotrexate can cause problems, so intake of the drug and the effect it is having needs to be monitored.

Before you start treatment it is possible that the doctor will want you to undergo a liver biopsy to ascertain the state of your liver. Under local anaesthetic a tiny piece of your liver is removed for examination. This is not a particularly uncomfortable procedure, but you will probably be kept in hospital overnight. You will almost certainly also be asked to have a blood test.

If you are put on Methotrexate you should have regular blood tests to keep a check on the condition of your liver and blood cells and your doctor may advise liver biopsies from time to time.

As you know, alcohol is bad for the liver. If you consume it while you are on Methotrexate you are greatly increasing your chances of damaging your liver. The odd glass of beer or wine occasionally should not harm you but it is best to do without it altogether.

The drug can affect the blood cells. Methotrexate works on the bone marrow which produces blood cells. It can reduce the amount of both red and white blood cells that the body makes. A reduction in the amount of red blood cells in your body can make you anaemic and chronically tired. A reduction in white blood cells makes you more prone to infection. Regular blood tests allow doctors to monitor the amount of red and white blood cells in your body.

Another possible side effect is mouth ulcers. This is not a good sign and may be an indication that you have over-dosed on Methotrexate. You must contact your doctor immediately if this occurs.

Sometimes people experience indigestion, stomach upsets or bowel problems when they are on this drug. If these problems persist you should contact your doctor.

Obviously, a drug as powerful as this cannot be taken during pregnancy. Methotrexate can damage the unborn baby. If you are pregnant you must not take this medicine and if you are thinking of trying for a baby you have to make a decision as to which you are going to do first. If you decide to go on Methotrexate, be very vigilant about contraception. It is also important to wait for a while after treatment is finished before allowing yourself to conceive. Three periods after the end of treatment is usually recommended.

Although not a great deal is known about the effects of Methotrexate on male sperm, it is advisable not to father a child while you are taking it. Again, it is considered best to wait three months after terminating treatment.

Another important thing to know about Methotrexate is that it does not mix with some other drugs. These include some medicines prescribed for heart disease, epilepsy, some antibacterial drugs, retinoids (prescribed for the treatment of psoriasis, see page 47), some non-steroid anti-inflammatory drugs (NSAIDs) as well as aspirin. So you really do need to check with the doctor if you are on any other medicine at all. And as some of the drugs Methotrexate does not mix with are ones that are bought over the counter, you need to be very careful about reading the label to see what the active ingredient is. If you are in any doubt, contact your GP.

Methotrexate is often prescribed for treating pustular psoriasis (also called palmar planter), generalized pustular psoriasis and psoriatic arthritis. Treatment can be for six months but it can take much longer to bring these serious conditions under control. Sometimes Methotrexate is given by injection.

· *The Retinoids* ·

This treatment for psoriasis was invented in the mid-1970s. Retinoids are related to vitamin A which is known to be important in the healthy functioning of the skin. Vitamin A promotes normal growth as well as good teeth and strong bones in children. It also helps to protect against infection.

The first retinoid tablet to be used for psoriasis was etretinate with the brand name of Tigason. This has now been superseded by acitretin which is the generic name for Neotigason. Neotigason reduces the production of keratin which is the protein that forms on the outer layer of the skin and gives it the thick, horny appearance.

These tablets are usually taken daily with a meal. Retinoids are also sometimes effectively combined with PUVA (a form of ultra-violet) treatment.

The main problem with this drug is the side effects. These can include dry, cracked lips which can become quite sore if they are not kept moisturised. There is also a drying of the inner lining of the nose and some patients experience sore eyes. Your doctor can give you drops for the nose and eyes to help to counteract this effect and vaseline works well for the lips. Thinning of the hair or even hair loss producing bald patches can be quite extensive. All of these side effects cease when treatment stops.

When this treatment first became available, an elderly lady who had taken part in the trials contacted the Psoriasis Association. She told them that her hair had fallen out during the treatment but grew back when the treatment stopped. She was delighted because she said that her hair was much nicer now than it had ever been. It had always been very straight (which she didn't like) but it had grown back wavy and a lovely shade of silver. However, a change in your hair type is by no means guaranteed!

Retinoids can also inflame the liver (but this is usually mild and does not normally give cause for concern) and raise the level of cholesterol in the blood. So, as with Methotrexate, regular blood tests need to be taken while you are on this treatment. Taken over a period of several years retinoids can also make changes to your bones. So you may need to have X-rays, now and again, to monitor this.

Retinoids can badly damage the unborn baby in pregnant women so it is imperative that if you are pregnant you do not take Neotigason. (Nor should you take large doses of vitamin A.)

If you are wanting to start a family it is important to think very carefully about whether or not to take retinoids. Since traces of the medicine remain in the body for two years, you will have to postpone pregnancy for a good two years after you have terminated treatment. That may seem too long. And during that time you will need to be very assiduous about contraception.

Retinoids do not seem to affect male sperm so these cautions do not apply to male patients.

Having given you the bad news it also should be said that many patients have experienced very good results with this treatment. A member of The Psoriasis Association reported in *The Journal of the Psoriasis Association* (Issue 69, 1995) that after more than 40 years of treating the condition to no real effect, Tigason (the drug which preceded Neotigason) had changed his life. He said that getting the dose right had been critical – too much had irritated the skin and two little hadn't worked. On a dose of 35mg a day he was experiencing virtually no scaling although the psoriasis lesions could be seen as faint red blemishes.

The side effect this patient reported was an initial drying of the mouth and nasal passages which soon passed and he had noticed that his skin was generally more fragile than before but this did not affect the healing process.

· *Cyclosporin* ·

This is a fairly new drug treatment for severe psoriasis. Cyclosporin is used in the main for transplant patients as it suppresses the rejection of transplanted organs. It can also be very effective in treating psoriasis.

Cyclosporin is an immunosuppressive drug which works by dampening down strong allergic and immune reactions. It also has anti-inflammatory properties. Any drug that suppresses the immune system should not be taken lightly.

People who have any serious infections, or may be suffering from cancer or who have had cancer in the past are not advised to take this drug. People who have a history of kidney disease, liver disease, high blood pressure, diabetes or high blood cholesterol may not be prescribed Cyclosporin. Pregnant women will also not be prescribed this drug.

Cyclosporin is taken orally in capsule or liquid form. The higher the dose the more effective it is in improving the skin but, equally, the more likely are there to be side effects. Perhaps the most worrying side effect is that it can reduce the efficiency of the kidneys, and taken over a period of time, this damage may be irreversible.

Like Methotrexate, Cyclosporin does not mix with some medicines. These include the non-steroid anti-inflammatory drugs (NSAIDs), some antibiotics, some anti-fungal treatments and some drugs for epilepsy.

Obviously, it is important to be monitored when taking this drug and, if you are on it, you will almost certainly be in the care of a dermatologist or dermatology clinic.

· *Hydroxyurea* ·

Like Methotrexate this drug is used as an anti-cancer treatment. With psoriasis it is used to stop cells growing too quickly. It is used if the psoriasis does not respond to other forms of treatment.

· *Non-Steroidal Anti-inflammatory* · *Drugs (NSAIDs)*

These are often used to treat psoriatic arthritis. They relieve stiffness, pain and inflammation of the bones and joints. They are called 'non-steroidal' to differentiate them from the corticosteroids described later on in this chapter. Corticosteroids also reduce inflammation.

NSAIDs work by blocking the production of prostaglandins. These are chemicals which are released by the body following injury and they produce the pain and the swelling. NSAIDs do not cure the condition, but in reducing the stiffness and swelling, they can make the injured joints easier to move and therefore more functional.

Different NSAIDs suit different people and you may need to go back to the doctor until you find one that suits you. Most of them are rapidly absorbed and short-acting. This means that the effects of the drug are experienced quite soon after you have taken them, so you should notice some relief within about an hour or so. However, the effects do not last longer than a few hours so you may be taking the pills several times a day to maintain the effect.

Side effects include indigestion and nausea. NSAIDs can sometimes cause bleeding in the stomach and should be avoided by people who have had peptic ulcers. They are not recommended for pregnant women or nursing mothers. People with liver or kidney abnormalities may also not be prescribed these drugs.

· *Sulphasalazine* ·

You may know this drug under the brand name of Salazopyrin. It is more commonly used to treat ulcerative colitis and Crohn's disease, both of which are conditions in which the bowel is inflamed. But sulphasalazine is also sometimes used to treat psoriatic arthritis as well as rheumatoid arthritis. The dose used to treat arthritis is very much lower than is used to treat bowel disease.

Nausea and loss of appetite are side effects that are more commonly experienced on higher doses of the drug that are not normally given for psoriatic arthritis. Most sufferers are prescribed a specially coated formulation of the drug. The prescription will carry the letters 'EN' which stands for 'Enteric Coated'. This coating minimises side effects.

Some people may find that their urine changes to a much more yellow or orange colour, but this is nothing to worry about.

Doctors usually recommend that you ensure a good fluid intake while you are on this drug.

· *Corticosteroids* ·

Systemic corticosteroids are very rarely prescribed for psoriasis. The two main reasons being that the side effects are worrying and that when treatment is stopped the condition returns, sometimes in a more severe form than before. However, if the psoriasis is so bad that the patient is seriously ill, this form of treatment may be considered to get the condition under control. When that has been achieved doctors can then look at other possible therapies.

Taken internally the drug can make you put on weight and give you a 'moon face' appearance. It can raise your blood pressure and your chances of getting a peptic ulcer. Taken for long periods it can thin the bones which can make you more prone to osteoporosis.

In providing the body with an increased amount of artificial cortisone (the hormone that helps the healing process), these steroids suppress the body's own cortisone-producing mechanism. The body is getting all it needs from elsewhere (the tablets) and can stop producing its own. This can have serious consequences in the case of an accident or injury. Normally, in these circumstances the body would go into over-drive and produce extra amounts of cortisone to aid recovery. If you have been on a medium-to-high dose of steroids for some time this is not likely to happen. So you have to take more artificial steroids in these circumstances to help heal the injury.

This is why it is so important to carry a card saying you are on steroid tablets. If you are in an accident, medical staff will know that they may have to give you steroids, along with anything else they may have to do, because your body will need them if you are to recover.

It is also very important to know that if you have been on steroid tablets for more than two to three weeks you have to come off them gradually and under medical supervision. The body needs time to adjust to the withdrawal of the cortisone and removing them suddenly could make you feel very ill.

You may not be prescribed these tablets if you have had tuberculosis, glaucoma or a peptic ulcer. If you suffer from diabetes, depression or osteoporosis it is unlikely that you will be prescribed systemic corticosteroids.

Please note that the side-effects stated above apply to systemic steroids and not to those applied topically.

5

SUNLIGHT AND ULTRA-VIOLET LIGHT

Many people with psoriasis find that sunlight has a beneficial effect on their condition. A sunny day gives most of us a psychological lift but it is more than that with psoriasis. Sunlight can speed up the healing process but only if it is treated with caution. Sunburn can make psoriasis worse.

The energy of the sun is radiated in different wavelengths. You can see some of these wavelengths in the colours of a rainbow. You may have noticed that these colours are red, yellow, green, blue, indigo and violet. Beneath the blue and violet colour is a wavelength that is not visible to the naked eye. This is ultra-violet light. And it is this wavelength of the sun's energy that affects the skin and, of course, psoriasis.

Ultra-violet contains quite a large band of light and can itself be divided into three groups: A, B and C. UVA is the nearest to visible light. On its own, UVA has very little effect on the skin, apart from producing suntan, but it is used to treat psoriasis. Patients are given medicines known as psoralens which make UVA treatment more effective. This is known as PUVA and is explained on pages 55–6.

The middle range of the ultra-violet band, UVB, is the one that has the most effect on our skin. It is the one that produces sunburn if we overdo it and it is also the one that brings about the improvement in psoriasis. UVB has to be administered under supervision, usually in a hospital physiotherapy department.

So, UVB is the burning wavelength of sunlight and UVA is the tanning wavelength.

There are some patients whose psoriasis is not improved by sunlight. It is important to notice if this applies to you. If it does, keep out of the sunlight or at least cover up because it could make your psoriasis worse.

UVC is a wavelength that is actually quite harmful to all living creatures but fortunately it doesn't get into the earth's atmosphere. The holes in the ozone layer have led to concern that UVC may be getting through but there is no evidence that this is happening yet.

· *Sunbathing* ·

If you find that sunlight helps your psoriasis there is no reason why you should not sunbathe, *providing you take it carefully and are aware of the fact that natural though sunlight may be, it is not without its side effects.* Sunbathing to improve your skin condition is known as Heliotherapy.

The skin protects itself from the sun by increasing pigmentation. So you turn brown. People with darker skin have a higher natural pigmentation than people with fairer skin. This is why they are able to withstand more sunlight. But even dark-skinned people will burn if they stay too long and unprotected in ultra-violet light.

Apart from the fact that sunburn can make your psoriasis worse, it can also increase the risk of getting skin cancer. But that's not all. Ultra-violet light can damage the collagen found in the dermis. Collagen gives the skin its pliability and elasticity. As we get older we have less collagen and this is what makes the skin appear more wrinkled. Over-exposure to the sun can reduce the skin's elasticity and make you look wrinkled earlier than you otherwise would.

So sunbathing can help your psoriasis. It can also be relaxing and enjoyable but it needs to be monitored so that you do not burn. Once your psoriasis has cleared, stop sunbathing. There is no advantage to continuing this self-help treatment. Extra sun will not prevent the psoriasis coming hack. Too much sunbathing may make the psoriasis more difficult to treat if it does return.

There are some medicines that make your skin extra sensitive to sunlight. Some antihistamines can do this, as can drugs taken for arthritis and other conditions. Also there are ointments and creams that can have this effect. If you are on any medication check with your doctor that it does not interact with sunlight before you go out in the sun as you could experience an adverse reaction. Antibacterial substances in special soaps as well as perfumes and cosmetics can also make the skin more sensitive to the sun.

If you are on PUVA or UVB treatment you must not sunbathe as you could suffer serious sunburn.

Here are some pointers to successful sunbathing.

- Get your skin gradually used to the sun. In spite of all the warnings some people still seem to enter into some sort of competition to see who can tan first as soon as the sun makes its appearance. Skin that has been covered all through the winter needs to be treated with great caution when it is first reintroduced to the sunlight.

Depending on your skin type, start by sunbathing for only a few minutes for the first few days, gradually increasing the time day by day, providing that you haven't become sore or burnt. But don't sunbathe for more than an hour or so at any time. Apart from risking burning, remember that sun dries the skin and that is not particularly good for psoriasis. *In fact sunburn can make the psoriasis worse.* There is a form of treatment that allows you to sunbathe eventually for up to eight hours a day. This is in the Dead Sea in Israel and there are special reasons why it is possible in this location. The Dead Sea treatment is described later on in this chapter.

- Always use a sunscreen. Check that the one you have chosen is all right for psoriasis. You need to look out for the Sun Protection Factor (SPF). The higher the SPF the greater the protection. People with pale skin that tans with difficulty and then only slightly are likely to burn easily. They should use a sunscreen with an SPF of 15 or more. People with darker skins may be able to get away with a SPF 10 sunscreen but if in doubt it is better to go for one with a high SPF than risk burning with a lower one. Pharmacists can be very helpful in discussing which sunscreen is best suited to your skin and many have charts which indicate which SPF factor you should have according to your skin type. So it is worth talking to your pharmacist about this.

  You can always start your sunbathing with a high SPF sunscreen and then go on to a lower one as your skin becomes more resistant.

- Re-apply the sunscreen after you have been swimming even, if the sunscreen is water-resistant.

- Remove any of the psoriasis creams or ointments you may have applied before putting on the sunscreen.

· *UVB Treatment* ·

Many patients who receive light treatment for psoriasis have UVB treatment. This is similar to PUVA treatment explained below but without the use of psoralens. As has already been stated, ultra-violet B is the shorter wavelength of light that has the most effect on our skin. It can be very effective in treating psoriasis but can also burn the skin if it is not carefully monitored.

People receive the treatment either as in-patients as part of a combination therapy like the Ingram regime explained in Chapter Three, or as out-patients in hospitals. Patients usually step into special cabinets which include the UVB lamps and they stand in these for the duration of the treatment. How long you spend in the cabinet depends on your skin type and the severity of the condition, but of course you start with a short period of time and gradually build this up as the skin gets more used to the treatment.

People wear specially tinted glasses or goggles to protect their eyes during their time under the lamps. They may also wear underwear to protect the genital area and breasts. If you are receiving UVB treatment you should not sunbathe as this increases the chances of getting sunburnt. For this reason people are not given this treatment prior to going on holiday in a warm, sunny location.

A few hospitals have a new type of UVB treatment which uses a narrow band of this light which is thought to be more effective, but this is not yet widely available.

· *PUVA Treatment* ·

As we discussed earlier on in this chapter, UVA light has very little effect on the skin. However, there are certain chemicals found in some plants that enable the skin to respond to this wavelength. These are called psoralens. Hence the name PUVA. This treatment has been found to be effective with common plaque psoriasis, pustular psoriasis and guttate psoriasis but is usually only offered when the condition is severe. It is an expensive treatment and the risks and side effects also have to be taken into consideration.

PUVA treatment is always given in hospitals as it has to be adapted to the individual and very carefully monitored. Also psoralen tablets are only available from a dermatologist.

Psoralens in tablet form take about two hours to be absorbed. So you will need to take them two hours before treatment. These tablets can make you feel sick or nauseous. If this is the case the dermatologist may switch to topically applied psoralens.

Some hospital departments may use psoralen in a liquid form. This may be applied directly on to the psoriatic patches or, if the psoriasis covers a large part of your body, you may be asked to have a bath in which some psoralen solution has been added. Both these latter methods are quicker in that you will probably only have to wait half an hour before having the UVA. Topically applied psoralens have been found to be just as effective as the tablet form.

You then step into a cabinet which incorporates the PUVA lamps for treatment. If the psoriasis is on your hands or feet, there are smaller devices which are used to treat just those parts of your body.

The length of time you stay under the lamps varies from person to person, but you will start with a few minutes and build up gradually. It is unlikely that you will spend any longer than 20 minutes under the lamps in any one session.

The dark tinted glasses or goggles you have to wear during the treatment are absolutely essential. The psoralens affect the lens of the eye, making them more susceptible to damage by the UVA light. You need to keep these glasses on from when you take the psoralen tablet to when you turn the light off when you go to bed that night. If you don't do this you run the risk of developing cataracts or damaging your eyes in other ways.

The goggles you use for the treatment will be supplied by the hospital but the tinted glasses you wear when you're not having treatment you will have to provide for yourself. It is important not to pick up any tinted glasses in the hope that they will work. Go to an optician and explain that you are having PUVA treatment and that you need glasses to cut out the glare of the light.

If you are having topical psoralens treatment you will not need to keep the glasses or goggles on all that time. You will probably only need to wear them during the treatment sessions themselves. In any event you need to check that the glasses or goggles are ones that block out UVA light.

You may experience a reddening of the skin soon after this treatment has begun. If it is accompanied by pain or soreness you will need to inform your doctor.

Remember that you should not sunbathe if you are receiving PUVA treatment. Nor should you expose your skin to any sunlight for some hours after receiving PUVA. If you are pregnant you cannot have PUVA so if you are already receiving this treatment or about to start, be extra careful with your family planning.

As with the previous sun treatments, PUVA can increase the chances of developing skin cancer. So you really do need to check out your skin regularly for any possible growths. This is the case even if you have had treatment some time in the past. If you notice a lump or a growth, contact your doctor immediately. Caught early, skin cancer is very treatable.

· PUVA Baths ·

This is the same treatment as above except that instead of taking a psoralen tablet you will be asked to take a bath to which some psoralen solution has been added. This treatment is recommended when psoriasis is widespread. You usually only have to wait half an hour after having the bath before having the UVA. You will, of course, have to wear the specially tinted glasses or goggles. This is a quick and effective method with the advantage that since you are not taking the psoralen into the system, you are much less likely to experience side effects. But some patients find it irritates the skin and not all hospitals have Bath PUVA on offer.

· Climotherapy at the Dead Sea ·

The Dead Sea is the lowest place on earth. It is situated some 400 metres below sea level. This means that the sun's rays have to travel an extra quarter of a mile through the earth's atmosphere. During this journey, many of the harmful effects of the sun's radiation are filtered out effecting a change in the balance of the UVA and UVB rays. The longer UVA rays are more predominant.

This means that it is possible to be in the sun for much longer periods of time without the same risk of burning. Of course you have to get your skin used to the sun first or you may burn.

UVA light is much more gentle to the skin. It is, as already discussed, used for PUVA treatment with the addition of psoralens. The reason for using psoralens is to make the skin more sensitive to this band of sunlight. Part of the reason for this is time. You cannot sit in an ultra-violet cubicle for hours on end, day after day, waiting for the UVA to work. It would be too expensive and totally impractical, so the process has to be speeded up.

The Dead Sea treatment depends on natural sunlight with no added chemicals but you have to put in the time. However, the success rate is good, and there are no chemically-induced side-effects. This treatment also reports good results with patients who have psoriatic arthritis.

As well as the sun there is the Dead Sea itself. This is rich in minerals which include chlorides, magnesium, sodium, calcium, bromine, potassium, sulphates and bicarbonates. Part of the treatment includes bathing in the Dead Sea.

In addition to the sea and the sun is the prevailing atmosphere of the area. The air itself contains many of the minerals, including bromine, that are known for their relaxing properties. Bromine helps the nervous system to relax. People sleep a lot which is very healing. Relaxation is considered to be a very important part of the Dead Sea treatment.

One of the best known Dead Sea treatment centres is The International Psoriasis Treatment Centre (IPTC) at Ein Bokek. Under the auspices of the prestigious Hadassah Hospital in Jerusalem, IPTC has been offering treatments to psoriasis sufferers worldwide for some 20 years now.

The treatment is tailor-made to the individual. The extent and severity of condition varies from person to person and the Centre treats all forms of psoriasis, including psoriatic arthritis, with the exception of erythrodermic psoriasis. Four weeks is the recommended length of stay for most patients.

When a patient first arrives he or she is given an examination by a dermatologist and a programme of treatment is devised. Some patients whose psoriasis is open and bleeding will not be able to bathe in the Dead Sea until the condition improves. This is because bathing would be too uncomfortable. They will start with a bit of sunbathing as well as the application of any topical preparations that may have been pre-scribed. The sunbathing is taken very gradually. Some patients will only spend five minutes in the sun to begin with while others will be able to stay there longer.

The solarium at IPTC consists of two large areas of beach that are screened off from the public. This is because sunbathing takes place in the nude so that there is one sectioned off area for women and another for men. Bathing in the sea, however, is unisex and, of course, in bathing costumes.

Patients arrive in the morning to sunbathe. Usually all that is applied is a simple emollient, often baby oil. Sun blocks are not used as the idea is to get the sun into the skin and the baby oil prevents dry-ing. There are several open air showers for people to use to cool down from time to time and there are shaded areas for patients to sit, out of the sun, but still in the beneficial atmosphere.

By midday patients will be back in their hotel rooms resting until the afternoon when they can sunbathe and bathe in the sea. By the end of two weeks most patients spend between six to eight hours in the sun with two dips in the sea in the course of a day.

There may be other treatments in their programme, including sulphur baths and the application of black mud.

It may sound a like a bit of a holiday, but in fact the treatment offered is very focused and IPTC boasts a success rate of 87% to 90% of patients returning home at the end of their four weeks with their psoriasis almost or completely cleared. For most of these patients the condition will have been severe when they arrived. The treatment does not seem to work so well for people who have been using systemic steroids or retinoids for a long period of time.

There is an understanding and acknowledgement of the psychological aspects of psoriasis. Dr. Roman Gumon, a dermatologist at the IPTC explains: 'I ask people to give me a mark on a scale of one to 10 as to how their psoriasis affects them emotionally or psychologically. Zero means that they are not affected at all and 10 denotes that they are suicidal. Most people find themselves between seven to 10. Young people are almost always at the higher end of the score.'

Dr. Gumon believes that a very important part of the success rate of the clinic is the psychological healing that is on offer there. 'People come here having spent so much of their time stressed because of their psoriasis. They have been embarrassed because of the appearance of their skin. They may have felt ashamed of it. Here they are the same as everybody else. They can remove their clothes without feeling embarrassed.'

Being in the company of other psoriasis sufferers is an important part of the healing process. Patients can exchange views, share experiences, offer coping strategies as well as sympathy and understanding. It removes the feeling of being 'different' and isolated. The remission lasts on average for eight months after the treatment has finished. Patients are sent home with the advice to keep their skins moist, usually with the use of simple emollients.

Psoriasis often does recur but usually with less severity. Patients tend to stay better for longer. Dr. Gumon says this compares very favourably with conventional treatment at the Hadassah hospital where he also works. With traditional treatments the condition comes back more quickly and sometimes with greater severity, particularly if steroids or retinoids have been used.

The clinic has had good results with psoriatic arthritis as well as rheumatoid arthritis. Sometimes people with quite severe disability can achieve much more mobility in their joints. Much of this is achieved by bathing in the Dead Sea. The joints are inflamed and painful. The Dead Sea is salty, oily and warm. This encourages people to try moving joints and muscles which would otherwise be too painful. Bit by bit as more movement is achieved the patient becomes more confident and is able to push the flexibility still further. Psoriatic arthritis is also treated with sulphur baths, black mud and physiotherapy. The treatment in general, however, is the same for psoriatic arthritis as it is for psoriasis.

Many of the patients at the clinic are paid for by Sick Funds operating in Germany, Austria and Denmark. These countries pay all the expenses of their psoriasis patients to be treated at the Dead Sea. This may seem unusually generous but in fact the treatment at the Dead Sea clinics is much cheaper than in-patient hospital care. Dr. Gumon reckons that it costs the same to treat a patient for one week at the IPTC as it does to treat a patient for one day at, for instance, the Hadassah.

Sadly, the NHS are not currently offering Dead Sea treatment for psoriasis sufferers so if you want to try it, you will have to fund yourself. Very few people can afford to go rushing off to the Dead Sea every time their psoriasis flares. Some patients go to the IPTC on an annual basis while others go every two or three years.

If you have been going through a bad patch with your skin (or joints) and need a therapeutic break, the Dead Sea treatment may be well worth considering. But remember, it is not a cure.

The address of IPTC appears under Useful Addresses at the end of this book, as does the address of VIP Health Holidays who can quote prices, give advice and book the package for you. The clinic is open all the year round.

6

BODY PARTS

Psoriasis can affect virtually any part of the body. Not only can the treatment and daily care vary depending on the area affected, but so can the social and psychological implications. This chapter aims to examine the condition as it affects the different areas of the body. Since psoriasis of the scalp is so commonly experienced among sufferers, let's start with that.

· *The Scalp* ·

Everybody's scalp sheds skin cells. These are normally not particularly visible. In the case of psoriasis, where the scalp is inflamed, skin cells are produced in large quantities. These are thick and silvery and shed frequently on to the shoulders, making them much more noticeable.

Psoriasis of the scalp can be extremely uncomfortable. It is often very itchy and the psoriatic patches which are inflamed and sore can start to bleed if they are scratched or picked.

The condition is *not* caused by poor hygiene or hair care. Nor does psoriasis affect hair growth. If you notice your hair falling out at a much greater rate than normal during a period of psoriasis, don't worry about it. Once the psoriasis has healed, the hair will grow back as thick as it was before.

Scalp psoriasis can be very demoralising. The look of the dead skin cells on your clothes can make you feel embarrassed and it is not always easy to brush them off inconspicuously. Try wearing light coloured clothes whenever possible, particularly on the top half of your body. Dark colours, especially black, can make silvery scales very visible.

The itchiness is another big problem. Having an itchy scalp that you cannot scratch is very distressing. And you do have to resist scratching, not just because of the social implications but also because it inflames the condition and makes it worse.

Some foods, such as shellfish, may make you itch. Food colouring, flavour enhancers, such as monosodium glutamate (MSG), and food preservatives can have this effect on susceptible people. If you suspect your itchiness is triggered or made worse by some of the things you eat, keep a food diary. Write down every thing you eat or drink in the course of a month. Read the labels to note the ingredients. Also note down the state of your itch each day. You may make an important link. If no link emerges and your scalp is extremely itchy, your doctor may be able to give you something (probably antihistamines) to reduce the need to scratch.

Another problem is that the lesions can often appear in visible areas of the scalp. The forehead along the hairline is a common site. So is the temple, the nape of the neck and around the ears as well as the hair parting.

However, having said all that, try not to let the condition put you off getting out and about and doing the things you want to do. There is considered to be a strong emotional element in psoriasis. Although it may be an inherited condition of the immune system, very often it is an emotional event that triggers a first attack. In any illness a person's state of mind can make a big difference to how quickly they get better and how well they keep. Becoming isolated and depressed can aggravate the condition. Feeling positive about yourself and enjoying your way of life can put you in remission and, with luck, keep you there.

For every person who stares at the silvery scales on your shoulder there will be someone who responds to you as a vulnerable and courageous human being. In some ways, the condition can help you to sort out the wheat from the chaff in terms of human relationships. The most important point to bear in mind is that you have to dominate the condition and not allow it to take you over.

Here are some general pointers.

- Brush your hair with a natural bristle brush, not a synthetic one. Don't brush your hair too frequently and brush very gently. Don't make the scalp tingle.
- Avoid a hairstyle that requires grips, clips, headbands or hair ties of any sort. A style that means pulling your hair back tightly may also inflame the scalp and aggravate the condition. But there is no need to cut your hair short if you prefer the longer styles. It just means that you will have to spend more time looking after your hair, but this is the case whether or not you have psoriasis.

One young woman rang up the Psoriasis Association in great distress because she had always had long hair and loved it and now, because she had psoriasis on her scalp, she had cut it short. She felt that she had lost an important and extremely attractive part of herself. The stress of cutting off her hair had made her psoriasis worse. So, although short hair may be easier to manage, you do need to take into consideration how you will feel if you are used to long hair and you cut it short. Anything that makes you feel good and more confident is worth having, even if it requires more work.

- It is best to let your hair dry naturally, but if you do use a hair dryer, make sure that you don't use it on a hot setting and that it is not too close to your scalp.
- You can perm or colour your hair unless you have scratched your skin. If your skin is open, the colour can go in so it is better to wait until it has healed. Vegetable dyes are usually better tolerated than chemical ones.
- As with psoriasis on other parts of the body, you may find that sunlight helps the condition.
- Try to not wear tight fitting headgear. Close-fitting hats or scarves tied tightly to the head can make the scalp hot and itchy.
- Try not to pick or scratch the scalp as you will make it bleed.
- Keep your nails short and make sure there are no sharp corners. This way if you do scratch you will do the minimum harm. Filing your nails is better than cutting them as it leaves less sharp edges.

Treatment varies depending on the nature of the psoriasis on the scalp. Some people will find that they can keep it under control through regular use of a special shampoo. Others whose scalp has thick crusty patches, will need to use an ointment as well to loosen these crusts. Of course creams and ointments stay much longer on the scalp than shampoos.

When treating your head with an ointment, bear in mind that the scalp is porous and so a higher proportion of the preparation will be absorbed than would happen in other parts of the body. So use the treatment with care, particularly if it is a steroid one such as Betnovate scalp application. But you do need to make sure that all the affected areas are treated.

Carefully part the hair in several different places to make sure that you have access to the spots that you want to treat. You may find that you need someone else to do this for you.

The best time to treat your scalp is at night so that the preparation is absorbed while you sleep. Cover the pillow with an old sheet or towel to prevent it from becoming soiled. The next morning, gently brush or comb the hair to take out the scales that have loosened during the night. They should come off easily. Now gently shampoo your hair.

Coal-tar shampoos and ointments have been used successfully for many years to treat psoriasis of the scalp. There is a wide range of coal-tar shampoos available over the counter without prescription. The ointments can be messy and smelly. Dithranol is another effective treatment but it can alter the colour of your hair particularly if you are blond or grey. Ointments containing steroids can also work but they need to be used with caution. Dovonex scalp application is also widely used.

Preparations which may be mixtures of different active ingredients are often made up to dermatologists' instructions to produce a particular effect. Ready-made formulations are also available.

One such compound treatment is Unguentum Cocois Compound which is an ointment combining coal-tar, salicylic acid and sulphur in a coconut oil base. The sulphur and salicylic acid help to remove the scale, and the coconut oil, which is a moisturiser, melts at skin temperature and helps to spread the preparation through the hair and over the affected skin. Messy to use, this successful treatment for severe scalp psoriasis is available over the counter and is made by Bioglan Laboratories.

Other widely used coal-tar formulations include Alphosyl 2 in 1, Capasal and Psoriderm. All these are available without prescription.

· *Ears* ·

Psoriasis can develop in the insides of the ear canal. Scales may clog the opening and make you temporarily hard of hearing. Topical treatment applied with a cotton bud can often help. You will need to see your doctor about this.

You must be very careful when treating the ear canal. If you use cotton buds make sure that you do not insert them deeply into the ear canal as this can damage the eardrum. Also the cotton buds must be sterile to avoid introducing an infection. If it is itchy, never use hard or non-sterile objects to scratch the itch as you can do a great deal of harm. Be particularly careful if you are treating a baby or child.

Scale and ear-wax can be removed by washing out the ear but this must be done under medical supervision. In many GP surgeries the practice nurse is available to provide this service.

· *Face* ·

Facial psoriasis can be very distressing because it is so visible. Also some of the creams and ointments that you would use on other parts of the body are not acceptable on the face because they stain the skin or are obvious in other ways. For these reasons many patients use steroid creams to treat facial psoriasis and this is fine, providing you are aware that these creams should be used sparingly. Used over a long period of time they can thin the skin and facial skin is particularly sensitive. Remember that when you stop using steroid treatment the condition often returns – sometimes in a more severe form. However, facial psoriasis is often successfully treated with cortisone (steroid) creams. But do see your doctor. He or she may have other treatments on offer.

Keep your face well moisturised and clean. Be sure to dry it gently after you have washed.

Women may find wearing a thick foundation good for camouflage purposes. Some beauty therapists can offer good advice free of charge, providing you buy their cosmetics, of course!

Many companies offer good cover-up make up. Almay, Avon, Boots, Clinique, Max Factor and ROC are some of the companies that produce good cover-up foundation in a variety of skin tones that can be used by women, men and children of all races. Some of these are waterproof which is useful if you are swimming. Some include sunscreen.

Obviously, you need to get the scaling off your face before applying the foundation.

If you have a bad problem with facial psoriasis, you can ask your doctor to refer you to the Red Cross. They offer a service for people with severe psoriasis who would like to learn camouflage techniques. Your skin colour is matched with specially formulated camouflage creams which have a very high pigmentation – something like six or seven times the pigmentation that you get in ordinary make-up and hence a lot of covering power. You are shown how to apply the creams and how to make them waterproof so that you can swim with them on.

Most of the Red Cross volunteers who work in this field operate from clinics in hospitals or from the local Red Cross branch head-quarters. The consultation is free but contributions are welcome.

If you want to know more about this service get in touch with your local Red Cross branch headquarters and ask to speak to the Therapeutic Beauty Care Officer.

Men may find it best to avoid shaving foam, astringents and after-shave as the perfume or alcohol may aggravate the condition. Dry shaving, with an electric razor, is usually best and you might find that applying a moisturiser after you have shaved is helpful.

· *Feet* ·

Psoriasis that appears on the soles of the feet can be very troublesome. This form of psoriasis is known as pustular psoriasis or palmar planter psoriasis. Sore feet can prevent you from walking any distance, taking part in sport or dancing so can be depressing as well as painful. When the soles of the feet become inflamed they produce a layer of thick, dry, dead skin. As the skin cracks and splits it becomes sore. Also the cracks and splits allow germs easy access and this produces further inflammation.

You need to rest your feet to give the inflammation time to die down and the lesions a chance to heal. Your doctor will probably prescribe topical treatment. Don't be lackadaisical about using it.

In addition to the treatment prescribed by your doctor, here are some tips:

● Soaking your feet in tepid water to which some salt has been added may help to heal the lesions. Counteract the drying effect of the salt by putting a moisturiser on afterwards. Do this before going to bed each night, for five to 10 minutes. But be sure to dry your feet thoroughly before applying any moisturiser or prescribed topical preparation.

● Gently pat your feet dry. Don't rub hard or hurriedly as this can make them more sore.

● Wear socks, stockings or tights that are 100% cotton or, if that is not possible, make sure that they contain as high a proportion of cotton as possible. Cotton fabrics allow the skin to breathe whereas synthetic fabrics are more restrictive in this way. Many of the large stores and chain stores sell cotton socks, stockings and tights and there are many direct mail companies that specialise in cotton garments. Cotton-on, whose address appears under 'Useful Addresses', is one but there are many others.

Better than cotton socks is bare feet. So try to keep your feet bare whenever possible.

- Shoes should also allow the feet to breathe. Leather shoes with leather lining or absorbent inner soles are good in this respect. Plastic footwear, trainers or other shoes that make the feet sweat should be avoided.
- You may like to try bandaging the feet at night once you have applied the creams or ointments. This will ensure that the medication is well absorbed.

· *Hands* ·

Psoriasis on the palm of the hands is pustular psoriasis, also known as palmar planter psoriasis, but on the backs of the hands it is called common plaque psoriasis. So treatment for each may be different.

Psoriasis on this part of the body can be distressing because it is visible and sometimes incapacitating. Many patients are embarrassed by it and hand psoriasis can cause problems at work. There are some jobs that you will not be able to do such as manual work. Handling food may also present a problem even though gloves are usually worn. If you notice someone staring at your hands, try to pluck up courage to tell them that what you have is psoriasis and that it is not catching. That is probably all they are worried about.

Hand psoriasis can appear as the result of an allergic reaction, such as to nickel found in rings. Rubber gloves can sometimes cause problems, especially if worn for long periods of time. If you have psoriasis on your hands, take it seriously. Rest your hands and do as little with them as possible until the condition has cleared. This includes dry work such as knitting, sewing, ironing, carpentry, DIY and the like as well as wet jobs like washing and cleaning. If you have sore hands, using them constantly is likely to keep them inflamed and cracking and the condition can become chronic.

Your doctor may prescribe a topical preparation to clear the condition but, if impractical, a systemic treatment may be prescribed instead.

Here are some general guidelines in caring for your hands.

- If soap irritates the skin, use a soap substitute, particularly if you are constantly washing your hands. Dry your hands gently and thoroughly and moisturise them afterwards. Keep tubes of emollient by the sink and washbasins.

- Keep hand washing clothes or other items down to a minimum and whenever possible use plastic or rubber gloves with cotton linings. The same applies to washing your hair. Do not wear these gloves for more than 20 minutes at a time. Wash them regularly in hot water.
- If you wear rings remember that the nickel in them could be a problem for you. The safest rings are those made with 18 carat gold, platinum and British Sterling silver. Never wash your hands when wearing a ring and don't keep rings on when you are doing housework. Rings need to be cleaned frequently. You can do this by soaking them overnight in 1 tablespoon of ammonia to 500 ml of water and then rinsing. Make sure you wear gloves when doing this to avoid getting the ammonia on your hands.
- Always wear gloves when using polishes, solvents and stain removers.
- If the psoriasis is on your hands and not your fingers, you may find that cutting the tips off the gloves gives you more flexibility in carrying out jobs.
- If you can, wash up in running water and always wear plastic or rubber gloves with cotton linings. If any water enters the glove, take it off immediately.
- In cold weather wear warm gloves, preferably leather ones with a cotton lining.
- Remember to rest your hands. Cracked, sore hands need rest, not work!

· *Folding Areas* ·

These include the armpits, under the breasts, under the chin, groin, navel, the skin behind the ears and between the fingers and toes. One of the most important points about these areas is that you need to be careful about drying them thoroughly after washing. If left moist, skin folds can chafe and become sore and injury to the skin can develop into psoriasis. The type of psoriasis that develops in these areas is known as flexural psoriasis. It is, as has been explained in Chapter Two, quite uncomfortable because of the soreness.

Tight-fitting clothes can irritate and cause sweating as can those made of synthetic fabrics. Underwear that fits tightly on the groin can cause problems as can close-fitting blouses and jumpers that hug the armpits. Try to wear garments that allow the skin to breathe. Cotton fabrics and loose fitting styles are a good bet.

· *Genitals* ·

Psoriasis can sometimes develop on this area of the body. With women it may be set off by excessive vaginal discharge as the result of a fungal infection called thrush. Or there may be other triggers like:

- Tight clothing that rubs
- Synthetic underwear
- Contraceptives, such as rubber sheaths, caps and spermicide jellies and creams
- Sanitary towels and tampons
- Rough toilet paper

Don't try to treat yourself. You do need medical help for this very sensitive area of the body.

If you have psoriasis in the genital area you may have to accept that you may not be able to have sexual intercourse until it clears. But it does not mean that you cannot have a sexual relationship. There are ways of being close and sexual that do not include penetrative sex.

If the woman has the condition she can lie with her partner and caress him to orgasm. It may be that the touching may not be able to be reciprocal but at least the sexual door is not closed. Equally, if the man has psoriasis and cannot have penetrative sex, he too can pleasure his partner and be pleasured by her without penetration taking place. This is very similar to the sexual enjoyment that many couples give each other after the birth of a baby when sex is also limited.

The most important aspect is literally to keep in touch and to be affectionate to each other. People with psoriasis need to feel loved and not rejected. But they also need to try to appreciate that feeling physically uncomfortable and emotionally demoralised can make them irritable and dismissive of their partners who may, in turn, feel rejected. In some ways it is up to the partner with psoriasis to take the sexual initiative – you know what you can and cannot do as well as what hurts and what doesn't. Your partner may be nervous of approaching you because he or she does not want to give you any more physical pain than you have already. Also he or she may fear that the approach will be met with rejection and you don't have to have psoriasis to want to avoid that.

Kissing, cuddling and holding hands are all loving gestures which make the other person feel wanted and desired. Try and stay in touch on an emotional and feeling level. Talk about how you feel and listen to your partner's feelings. This can often be a more intimate and loving way of relating to someone than sex. Intimacy is as much about sharing feelings as it is about making love. Being able to express your feelings to someone who cares can be a very healing experience and could well have a beneficial effect on your psoriasis.

· *The Joints* ·

Between five and 10 percent of people with psoriasis experience inflammation of the joints, known as psoriatic arthritis. For most people this means nothing more than one or two mildly aching joints, but for a few patients the condition is much more severe and can, in some rare cases, be disabling. It is essential to seek expert help in the early stages of psoriatic arthritis (or any other form of arthritis) to try to prevent the condition from deteriorating.

When a joint is inflamed, it swells and is sore. It is also usually warm to the touch. You may or may not find that psoriasis develops on the site of the inflammation. Sometimes it appears elsewhere. Rest is again the key to treatment, but the trouble is that very often the inflamed joint is the one you use most. If your work involves writing a lot or you are a seamstress, cook or housewife, you may find that it is a finger joint that becomes inflamed. A dancer or athlete may suffer inflammation of a joint in the foot.

Don't lift and carry if doing so is going to stress the inflamed joint. You will need to become more discerning about what you do and how you do it and this includes everyday tasks. Do you need to open that bottle, for instance? What effect is it going to have on your arthritic finger joint?

Many devices have been designed with arthritis sufferers in mind. With these, sometimes ingenious inventions, you can open bottle tops or turn taps with few problems and there are also kitchen gadgets and DIY appliances that have been developed for use by people with arthritis. Your doctor may be able to put you in touch with a local occupational therapist who can give you more information on this.

In any event, if you develop arthritis, you should go and see your doctor straight away and remind him that you are a psoriasis patient.

· *Legs* ·

Psoriasis on the calves or shins can be very itchy. Swollen or varicose veins on the legs can make the condition worse. Women and overweight people are more prone to varicose veins. If you have swollen or varicose veins, wear support stockings, tights or bandages during the day. Do not stand on your feet for long hours. Rest with your legs raised as much as possible. Topical preparations can be very helpful in reducing the inflammation and controlling the itch.

· *Nails* ·

Psoriasis can appear on toe nails as well as finger nails and it is quite troublesome to treat. Topical treatments can be messy to apply and difficult to keep on. The effects of psoriasis on this part of the body can vary from person to person. Finger nails tend to be pitted, with dents and rough patches appearing on the surface. Sometimes the nail can become discoloured or it can separate slightly from the nail bed. If your nail has gone a green/black colour it may have become infected and you'll need to see your doctor to get it treated.

Toe nails with psoriasis tend to get thick rather than pitted.

- Keep your nails very clean. Bits of dirt that accumulate between the underside of the nail and the finger can introduce infection to any psoriatic lesion that you scratch.
- Nails should be kept well manicured. You may find nail clippers easier to use than scissors. Although nails should be short, be very careful not to cut them so short that they are uncomfortable. Take time over manicuring.
- Dry your nails thoroughly after washing your hands.
- Use nail varnish to hide the nail blemishes. You may find it best to use a base first to reduce the effects of any colour.

· *Joyce* ·

Joyce first had psoriasis when she was 31 years old and the mother of two young children. She knew what it was because she comes from a family of psoriasis sufferers. Joyce is one of nine children. Her younger sister had it severely as a child and young adult and two of Joyce's brothers have psoriasis. She has cousins and nephews with the condition, but neither of her parents suffered from it.

Joyce's psoriasis has changed over the years. It first came on the scalp and hairline and spread to other parts of her body. There was a period when the scalp psoriasis was very severe as she describes below. Now at 54, Joyce's psoriasis is mainly flexural. Here is her story.

I went to a dermatologist who gave me treatments to use at home. I treated it for six weeks with salicylic acid and coal-tar scalp treatment. I used to put the ointment on my head every night and get up the next morning to wash it out. And then I would have to set my hair. You didn't blow-dry in those days. You had to put it in rollers and sit under a hair dryer and I used to do all that before taking the children to school and going on to my own part-time job.

The ointment would go all over the bedclothes and all over anything I wore. But after six weeks it improved quite a lot.

But then when we moved to Wales to run a guest house my psoriasis came back with a vengeance. It was very hard work and I was very tired and lonely. I'd left my family and friends behind and I was very homesick. I think that made it worse. My psoriasis has never cleared completely since then even though we returned to my home town four years later.

The psoriasis on my scalp was really bad years ago. It was disgusting. My hair used to fall out. The scales were very thick on the head. I used to put the ointment on and rinse it off later, but as my scalp started drying out it became so taut that it felt as if I had an elastic band around my head all the time. It made me feel physically ill.

Sometimes I'd put the ointment on and as I combed it through big lumps of scale would come off and my hair would break and come out with it. It fell out everywhere. I could see the scales sticking out in my hair and people would comment. They'd tell me I'd got this big piece of white stuff on my hair and I'd say that it was only my psoriasis.

It looked dreadful with big lumps of skin falling off my head. I'd never be able to get dressed up or anything. And that lasted for months. It was depressing. It doesn't do much for your ego, your sex life or anything. You feel so unattractive. But that was years ago. Fortunately, it's never been like that since.

I'm lucky in the sense that my psoriasis has never been on my hands or my feet. It has been flexural psoriasis for a long time now. With flexural psoriasis the skin doesn't shed. It is sore and red and it splits. It is under my arms and under my bust and in the groin area. It is also behind my ears and inside my elbows – all the body folds. As long as I don't take my clothes off I'm okay. I can cover it up and most of the time people probably wouldn't know that I had psoriasis. Until this year my legs and arms were not a problem.

I remember going to Malta on a family holiday one year. It was terribly hot. Normally I would never strip off. I would put my swimsuit on with a sundress on top and then I would go down to the side of the water, take off my sundress and jump in before anyone had time to see anything. And I wouldn't come out of the water if anybody was there. But in Malta I tried sunbathing and I noticed some young Maltese girls were pointing at me and they were obviously talking about me.

I think the worst part of psoriasis is the embarrassment of it all. You haven't got the freedom to take your clothes off and sunbathe or go *swimming like other people. You can't use communal changing rooms in shops and places like that. It's the ignorance of people who don't understand that gets to you.*

My daughter was getting married earlier this year. My skin was in a terrible mess. It was all over me. I hadn't been so bad for years. I went to see the consultant and asked to be put on a course of treatment to get me better and more presentable for the wedding. I went on a course of PUVA treatment from April to August.

In the past I've had the psoralen tablets but this time I had psoralen baths. It was much better. You don't need to mess about wearing the dark glasses for hours afterwards. You soak in the bath for 10 minutes, have the sunlight treatment and then shower it off. I started by going three times a week and then it was reduced to twice a week.

I stopped treatment on the week of the wedding. I had a suntan and my skin was clear. I looked great!

I think a lot depends upon what is happening in your life. I definitely think that my psoriasis is irritated by stress. As a family we don't cope very well with stress and responsibility. When we have to take on responsibility we do it, but we're not laid back about it. We are a very highly strung family – all of us. Yet only some of us have psoriasis and I have often wondered why.

7
DEPRESSION

Having a chronic illness like psoriasis can colour many aspects of your life, particularly if the condition is severe. A number of studies have been carried out by researchers to investigate the psychological effects of psoriasis on its sufferers. Psoriasis patients reported difficulties in establishing social contacts and relationships. Some mentioned embarrassment and others felt the need to wear clothes that covered their lesions.

The authors of one study found that 50% of sufferers believed that psoriasis inhibited their sexual relationships. 11% reported that they would avoid having children in case their offspring developed psoriasis. Another study reported that 64% of sufferers avoided public places such as restaurants.

There is little doubt that for many people the worst part of having psoriasis is the social isolation it can cause. One patient said that he was afraid to leave his house because of the stares and the unkind remarks directed at him.

Many psoriasis patients mentioned sexual problems caused directly by the condition. It can be difficult to feel sexual when your skin is sore and your morale low. But it's even worse when your partner is put off by the way you look. One man whose psoriasis suddenly flared up after he was married said that it had had a disastrous effect on his sex life. The psoriasis was on his genitals, as well as other parts of his body. This not only made penetration or touching in that area painful sometimes, but his wife could not bear to be penetrated by him. She could not stand the prospect of his skin coming off inside her.

A young and pretty 21-year-old girl whose psoriasis was mainly on her body became nervous about embarking upon relationships with men. She worried that if the friendship became physical to the point where she had to take off her clothes, the man in question would recoil from the sight of her body.

If you can get over the social distancing, the psoriasis itself becomes more bearable. As one patient put it: 'Everybody likes to be loved. We all like to have friendships. Everyone likes to feel good when they're with somebody that they care about. When you haven't got that there is a vital spark out of your life'.

As you read through some of the stories in this book you will see that a high proportion of psoriasis sufferers do not swim or sunbathe in public places. Many do not wear clothes that reveal their bodies. For others the limitations can been even more severe.

· *Disability* ·

It seems that there is not always a direct correlation between the severity of the psoriasis and the disability, distress or depression experienced. Disability seems to have more to do with how psoriasis affects the sufferer's life rather than how extensive the condition is.

Where the condition appears on the body is the main factor in determining the extent of the disability experienced and the resulting distress.

If someone has psoriasis on their face and hands as well as other parts of their body, it might be better to concentrate on clearing their face and hands and not worry so much about the rest.

Treatments for psoriasis can themselves be disabling. If you have to turn up for UVB or PUVA therapy three mornings a week and the hospital is at the other end of town, it is going to take a great deal of time. This may threaten your job or, if you are a mother of young children, it can be extremely stressful. So it might be better to look at the treatment from the point of view of what is going to improve the everyday living of the particular sufferer rather than just concentrate on clearing up lesions.

Dr. Jonathan Barker, consultant dermatologist with the St. John's institute of Dermatology, advocates this. 'When you are treating people, you tailor the treatment to the patient, he says. 'The goal is to improve the patient's quality of life. Every patient has a different expectation of their treatment. Some people have very bad psoriasis but are prepared to put up with it, whereas others have very little psoriasis but hate having a single spot. Most people are somewhere in the middle. What we aim to do is to find out what the patient wants from the treatment and we go along with that'. This sometimes means asking the patient to choose the areas they most want to clear and concentrating on that.

But even with the best treatment in the world, there are times when sufferers feel depressed. This is inevitable for anyone suffering from a condition that keeps recurring. But for the most part these feelings pass as you get on with your life. Good things happen; maybe the skin clears considerably and you enter a more positive spiral.

However, there are times when depression may deepen. An accumulation of disappointments and a skin that is difficult to treat can be very wearing and it is not always easy to feel cheerful or positive about the future. If you then add to this an unhappy experience, like, for instance, a bereavement, you can become very depressed and enter a downward spiral which may be difficult to stop without outside intervention.

Sheila's story, which appears below, illustrates this point. She had, with great resilience, put up with being ill and having to face not being able to pursue the career of her choice. But it took her mother's death to trigger the depression. 'I realise now that there had been something brewing for a long time,' she says. 'I was very close to my mother and when she died I went to pieces.'

But it doesn't have to be a bereavement or a trauma that initiates depression that needs treatment. Sometimes you cannot 'just pick yourself up'. This is true of most illnesses. Take the example of viral infections. Normally you get a runny nose, sore throat, headache, maybe a temperature and you go to bed, drink plenty of hot drinks, take some painkillers and in a few days you are back on your feet again. But there are other times when the infection takes more of a hold and if you don't contact the doctor and get it treated, you are likely to become more ill with, perhaps, pneumonia, bronchitis or some other secondary infection.

It's the same with depression. Most of the time you can lift yourself out of it and carry on, but sometimes you cannot, and you may need to see a doctor or try one of the talking treatments described in the next chapter. As with any other illness, the important thing with depression is to understand what it is and when and how it needs to be treated.

· *Recognising Depression* ·

Most of us get depressed from time to time. Nothing seems to be going right and we feel down in the dumps, inadequate and generally fed up. There may be a trigger to these depressed feelings like a disappointment, or a loss or it may be a feeling that arrives from nowhere. But a few days later the mood changes, either of its own accord or something happens to cheer us up. Most people experience this kind of depression from time to time and cope with it in different ways. Some will talk to friends or relatives whose support pulls them through a rough patch. Others might find that throwing themselves into a hobby or sporting activity lifts the gloom and allows them to see things in a more positive way.

But depression can sometimes be much more severe than that, so much so that it dominates the sufferer's life, rendering him or her incapable of doing very much at all. In this case, depression is an illness. And just like any other illness it needs to be taken seriously and treated. In the same way as telling someone with severe psoriasis to 'snap out of it' is likely to do nothing for their skin apart from, perhaps, make it worse, clinical depression cannot be cured by being told to 'pull yourself together'.

Mild depression can often be overcome with self-help strategies like the ones described later on in this chapter. But for more severe depression outside expert intervention is often required which can be in the form of talking treatments or through a short course of drug treatment.

People are beginning to be less embarrassed to say that they feel depressed and doctors are becoming more alert to the symptoms of the condition and are consequently better at diagnosing it. They are also more versatile in treating it. Many GP surgeries these days have counsellors and psychologists who can offer treatment to depressed patients.

In 1992 the Royal College of Psychiatrists and the Royal College of General Practitioners launched a joint 'Defeat Depression' campaign. It is an education campaign to inform the public as well as doctors how to recognise and treat depression. It seems that some of their work is paying off.

· *Symptoms* ·

Here are some symptoms of depression. You do not have to experience them all to be depressed, although the first one is fundamental. If you have been experiencing four or more of the other symptoms for two weeks or longer and there has been no particular trauma recently (like a bereavement), you may need to take your feelings seriously and realise that as they may not go away of their own accord, you should consider going to see your doctor.

- Loss of interest or pleasure in life. In mild depression you may experience good days and bad days, often with mornings and evenings being the worst times. In a more severe form the world seems very gloomy indeed with nothing to offer.
- Exhaustion. We all get very tired from time to time, but if you are constantly tired for no particular reason, it may be a symptom of depression.
- Sleep disturbance – either insomnia or sleeping too much.

- Loss of concentration. Being unable to read a page of a book you would normally enjoy without your mind wandering, or being unable to pay attention to what is going on around you could be caused by depression. This is often accompanied by poor memory and forgetfulness.
- Appetite changes. As a rule people suffering from depression eat very little and lose a lot of weight very quickly. Some people, suffering from mild depression, eat much more than they should and often the kind of food that will make them fat.
- Constant irritability, going off sex, loss of confidence, an inability to make decisions are all possible symptoms of depression. Most of us may find it difficult to decide what clothes to buy or which holiday to take, but with depression decisions such as whether to have tea or coffee, toast or bread or what pair of socks to wear become difficult.
- Feelings of guilt and worthlessness, agitation and panic.
- Suicidal thoughts. These are an extremely important sign that the illness needs expert help.

· *Treating Depression* ·

Given that depression is such a destructive and all-pervading illness, why do so many people not seek help to overcome it? An interesting explanation appears in the book *Depression and How to Survive it*, by Spike Milligan and Anthony Clare, published in paperback by Arrow priced £5.99. 'One of the major difficulties affecting those of us who get depressed is that because of our apathy, loss of hope, sheer misery, feelings of guilt and self-reproach, and disinclination to bother people with what seems to be a hopeless case, we just do not believe there is any point in seeking help'. Friends and relatives don't know how to help and may not even recognise the seriousness of the situation.

There are different ways of treating depression. The talking treatments outlined in the next chapter can be extremely effective. Long-term talking treatments can be expensive but they can also alter your perspective and enhance your life in addition to lifting the depression. Many doctors' surgeries offer the services of a psychologist or counsellor which may be available on the NHS.

Drug treatment with anti-depressants can also work well. Taken regularly, anti-depressants can start to lift the symptoms of depression in about two to four weeks. Treatment is usually continued for about six months afterwards, sometimes longer, depending on the severity of the condition as well as other factors. Side effects with anti-depressants can include drowsiness, constipation and a dry mouth but these usually only occur in the early stages of treatment and then subside. *Anti-depressants are **not** addictive.*

There is also self-help. Below are some pointers to helping yourself which you can do in addition to the expert help you may be receiving. If your depression is very mild, taking some of these suggestions on board may help to stop the depression getting a hold, becoming more severe and requiring outside help.

Talk! Keeping things to yourself is not a recipe for happiness, particularly if you have had bad news or suffered some serious setback or trauma in your life. Everyone needs someone they can talk to who will listen and not gossip. Talking is probably the best therapy and it is surprising how many people find it difficult to confide in anyone. Men, in particular, find it hard to have friends they can talk to about their feelings and fears. It is not uncommon for men to have male friends that they drink or watch sport with and women friends they confide in. But some men and, to a much lesser extent, some women have no-one they talk to.

It is surprising how much better you feel when you've had a long talk and a good cry with someone you trust. Knowing you have been heard can be a good way of starting the healing process. Don't turn yourself into a pressure cooker. Allow some of the bubbles to rise to the top and evaporate.

Eat! Food can seem very unappealing when you are depressed but you do need to keep to a nutritious diet. You don't have to make elaborate meals for yourself. Try and eat plenty of fresh fruit and vegetables which are full of vitamins. Getting ill can only make the depression worse.

Go out! It may be the last thing you want to do but try and find something to do outside the house each day. Going for walks will give you plenty of fresh air and exercise which will help you to sleep better. Going to the cinema or looking around the shops can take your mind off things and help you feel a bit better at least for a while.

Exercise! If you possibly can, try and do some kind of exercise. This will keep you fit. Rigorous exercise gets rid of the build-up of adrenaline and helps to reduce stress.

Sleep is not so important. Don't worry about not sleeping. Read a book, listen to the radio, watch television or do anything else that rests your body. You may drop off to sleep when you stop worrying about it, but if you don't, it doesn't matter.

Alcohol is not a good option. It may be tempting to drink to blot out feelings but the relief alcohol brings is very short-lived. In fact, alcohol is a mood depressant so is likely to make things worse in the long run. Using alcohol to block feelings resolves nothing. The hurt and unhappiness are still there and if you have been drinking heavily you may have the added problem of alcohol-dependency or addiction to cope with as well.

A good book on depression is *Depression: The Way out of Your Prison* by Dorothy Rowe. It is published in paperback by Routledge.

· *Sheila* ·

Sheila was born with psoriasis. It appeared when she was three days old and it has been with her, in one form or another, ever since. She is 32 years old and now has guttate psoriasis.

I don't have plaques at all. I have tiny red spots all over my body. On my face, from my neck upwards, I have very fine dry skin which comes off every morning. I literally peel off ear-shaped flakes which come off in large pieces. It is like removing a mask. They have got smaller over the years but when I was a little girl you could take sheets of it off in one piece. It leaves my skin very red and sore.

Until I was 13 I had hardly any hair and very thick scabs on the top of my head. Until last year I wore a wig.

My psoriasis has gone through various stages. When I was a little girl and until I was 16 it was very pustular and yukky. When I was a baby my mother used to have to put me in the bath with my vest still on because I was stuck to it. I must have been a disgusting child. What would really get me down was that I used to get a very pustular face and that was horrible. Fortunately my skin has got much drier over the years. I do still get pustules very occasionally on my nose but that is rare now.

When I was a child people stared at me. I think my mother probably suffered most because people thought I'd got burnt and she'd be accused of keeping me out in the sun too long. As a child you are very aware that you are different, especially with a skin complaint. People were a lot more ignorant then than they are now.

I was very ill when I was 16. I was sitting my exams at school and my skin got very bad. I suppose it was the stress. I kept piling on the steroids. I find that if you use steroids long-term you don't stop the psoriasis coming back. It will just come back 10 times worse and this was what was happening. My skin kept flaking off left, right and centre. It was hot to the touch and very red. I was throwing out a lot of heat. I lost control of my body temperature.

They took me into hospital and I suppose to get me back to being reasonably well quickly they put me on Methotrexate. I've never been able to come off it completely even though my skin is much better now. I'm on a very low dose, but while I'm on it, I can't have children.

I came out of hospital eight weeks later feeling very sore and fed-up. I was meant to be starting college to do a pre-nursing course, but I had been told that I couldn't do nursing because of my skin. I was very disappointed. I'd always wanted to be a nurse. But I've worked in a succession of old people's homes.

I thought I had come out of my childhood relatively unscathed, but it does catch up with you. I had a nervous breakdown after my mother died. I think it was cumulative. I was stressed and hassled with life in general.

I realise now that there had been something brewing for a long time. I was very close to my mother and when she died I went to pieces. First I was in a state of shock. Then I became very depressed. I had been studying for a year and my memory went. I couldn't remember anything I'd learnt. I now know that memory loss is a sign of severe depression but I did not know that then. I didn't want to work or have much to do with the human race. I just wanted to opt out. I had to give up my job and I spent most of my time on my boyfriend's farm.

Some time before my actual breakdown I'd been put on Prozac (an anti-depressant) which was very good initially. It works for about six months and then you have to come off it and try and do without it. I was on Prozac much longer than that and it ended up making me worse because it made me very debilitated and drowsy. I wasn't getting anything done or achieving anything. In the end I flushed the pills down the toilet. I'd been on them for nearly two years.

I have some very good friends and family and they saw me through that time until bit by bit I was able to build my life up again.

I am in a relationship with someone and it is a very loving and caring relationship but he doesn't actually want to settle down. Sometimes I wonder if it is because of my skin. I suppose it always will affect me in some ways.

You don't have as much confidence as you might. If something goes wrong you have a tendency to blame it on your skin, which is preposterous. You have to keep a very careful check on yourself so that you don't blame everything on psoriasis. And you have to try not to let it get you down too much.

Relationships are not easy. I look unusual with my skin. And with psoriasis you're aware that you are a bit different from other women. Consequently, you are afraid that your partner will meet somebody else. You always have that at the back of your mind.

When I was 16 I was too sore to be cuddled. I was raw and yukky. I wouldn't want anyone I care about to see me like that. So although I've never been as bad as that since, I'm always afraid that I may get to that stage. It worries me, so maybe in some ways it's a good thing that I'm single. But it's not the desired state.

8

PSYCHOLOGY AND TALKING TREATMENTS

People seem to fall into three categories when it comes to regarding the importance of the psyche in any given situation. There are those who think that everything is in the mind. This view was given credence by the 'there are no accidents' school of therapists who believed that the unconscious had a part to play in everything. So, if you tripped over the cat and twisted your ankle you were supposed to search your psyche for a deep and meaningful reason why. This fateful line of thought put a lot of people off considering the possibility of a psychological component in what might appear to be a practical problem or organic illness.

There are those who reject the psychological aspects of a situation. So they reject it entirely as 'psychobabble'.

In the middle are the majority of people who believe that there may be unconscious issues behind some of our problems but it is not the whole story.

With an illness like psoriasis that sometimes involves patients in taking drugs that have serious side effects, it seems worthwhile to examine the possibility that there may be an emotional or psychological component to the condition. We know that very often a trauma can trigger an attack. Is there a psychological problem that keeps it going? Or is part of the psoriasis a manifestation of an emotional or psychological conflict? With these questions in mind, let's have a look at some of the psychological issues that may be involved.

*Please bear in mind that this chapter is not trying to label psoriasis as a psychological illness. It has already been stated that patients inherit a predisposition to it and that doctors believe psoriasis may be caused by a malfunctioning immune system. What we are looking at here is the possibility that there may **also** be a psychological input.* This would be true of almost all the chronic illness that people experience including asthma, eczema, ulcerative colitis and irritable bowel syndrome.

If you look at psoriasis from the viewpoint of a psychotherapist, you may see it as an outlet for unexpressed emotions. It may be that the person has never been able to express hurt and anger and other negative emotions verbally and these bottled-up feelings are expressed through the skin.

Some psychotherapists see skin as the boundary between the inner being and the outer persona. A skin ailment may be seen as a way of making the inner and hidden emotions visible. And since skin is such an important part of a person, skin conditions are seen as a very heart-felt way of showing distress. Sometimes this distress is hidden and sometimes it is not. It is well known that students often have outbreaks of psoriasis or eczema at exam times. The anxiety of the exams is too much to handle and so it breaks out in the skin. Students often know that this is likely to happen and they expect it and prepare for it.

We all experience emotional conflict, upset or even trauma that we cannot handle with our normal coping mechanisms. Some of the pain of those experiences may remain buried in the psyche long after we have stopped agonising over the events. This can happen, for instance, when someone very close has died and we haven't been able to grieve properly at the time. We may carry the grief around in our unconscious and it is possible that some of those feelings of unhappiness then become expressed through illness.

Another theory is that an accident or trauma may be a release of something that happened much earlier in life in, for instance, babyhood where there are no words. For instance, a recent involvement in a car crash may have triggered psoriasis. People understand that car accidents are traumatic and you are able to talk about it and maybe even link the onset of psoriasis to it. But this accident may re-play another dramatic incident in your early childhood that you do not remember. You may have been dropped as a baby, for instance. You don't remember it or anything about it and you were certainly unable to talk it through, but the current event releases the memory of the early trauma into your unconscious. What enters consciousness is the stress factor.

Or the patient may be a person who has difficulty in handling conflict or confrontation. Take, for example, this situation. Sam is out with Jane whom he doesn't know very well but is anxious to impress. A complete stranger is very rude and belittling to Sam in front of Jane and he doesn't handle it well. He just shrugs it off, pretending he doesn't care but inside he wants to curl up and die. He also feels very angry with himself for not shutting the stranger up, or 'giving as good as he got'. He may feel that he let himself down and that Jane now thinks he is a wimp. This may stop him from furthering his friendship with Jane or he may push the incident to the back of his mind and carry on as if nothing happened.

Either way, the chances are that the anger, hurt and frustration will be lodged in Sam's unconscious and if he is a psoriasis sufferer, these feelings may be expressed through his skin. This is not a particularly unusual scenario. Most of us do not like confrontations and we don't deal with them the way we would like. If our handling of such a situation is far off our expectation of ourselves, the anger and frustration gets expressed in other ways. One of these ways can be illness.

Talking treatments can put some of these feelings into words. The British Association of Psychotherapists says: 'Psychotherapy can help by teaching understanding of the internal problems so that they are expressed in words rather than through the language of the body. This can give hope for change and resolution'.

The emotional problems of having psoriasis are, of course, linked with the psyche. *David*, whose story appears on pages 121–3, says that he was called a 'leper' by one of the customers in the bank where he was manager. This is not an unusual experience for psoriasis sufferers and is unlikely to pass by without emotional and psychological repercussions. *David* puts a brave face on it and takes his shirt off on a crowded beach and laughs when the surrounding area suddenly clears. But he says that the bravado is a cover for the hidden feelings of vulnerability that he carries inside. And the bravado embarrasses his wife.

For every *David* there are thousands of psoriasis patients who hide away, covering their skins because, not surprisingly, they cannot handle the stares, hurtful comments and rejection. One patient commented that you only look good if your skin is looking good and in this day and age when the feel-good factor seems to have been inextricably linked with how you look, it is hard to feel good about yourself if you are overweight, under-endowed or have a flaky skin. It is not surprising therefore that so many psoriasis patients suffer from depression at some time or another.

Tony says in Chapter Two (see pages 24–6) that talking is essential. When he gets depressed he drops in on a friend for a chat. Married to someone who has psoriasis and psoriatic arthritis, he observes that it is not always easy to talk to the person with the illness for fear of hurting them or being misunderstood.

This can also be true, at times, of talking to friends. It is sometimes much easier to talk to a stranger who doesn't know you, your family or friends than it is to talk to someone you know well. It doesn't matter what they think of you since they are not part of your world. And your secrets stay with them.

An open ear and sealed lips are on offer in talking treatments and it is the feelings of loneliness, emotional distress, poor self-image and lack of self-confidence that these treatments are good at addressing. Other bonus points are that there are no drug-induced side-effects and, when the treatments work, the effects are usually long-lasting.

A talking treatment is unlikely to change Sam from a retiring person to one who thrives on confrontation, but it could help him to express his feelings of sadness or anger verbally. It may well help him to see himself in a more positive light which would change many aspects of his life, including his health.

As has been explained in the previous chapter, talking treatments can be very helpful in treating depression.

Below is a brief description of some of the main talking treatments available, but there are many others and, if you are thinking of trying one, it might be worth getting to know a little bit about some of them before embarking on any particular one. It is also very important that you see a properly trained therapist in whichever field of therapy you choose. The addresses of the professional bodies of the therapies mentioned here appear in 'Useful Addresses' at the back of the book.

· *Psychotherapy* ·

Psychotherapists believe that the kind of person you are today is based on your childhood. This is not just a question of what experiences you had as a child but a mixture of many things. How you were brought up; what expectations your parents had of you, how they behaved towards you; your place in the family pecking order; the behaviour patterns you have unconsciously learnt from your parents and brothers and sisters; your experiences with friends and at school and so on. All this, together with the genetic characteristics you were born with, has made the individual that is you.

It is a psychotherapist's job to help you unlock some of these emotional doors and find the clues that will help you to understand why you behave the way you do. To carry on the theme of unresolved anger and inability to confront, it may be that in Sam's family people did not get angry. People didn't shout at each other. No-one lost their temper. Issues were resolved by punishments, people leaving the room, or isolating the 'trouble-maker', and so on. So Sam grew up with the belief that it was not done to express his anger verbally, and *he had to find some other way.*

Or, perhaps there was someone in Sam's household who had a terrible temper and when he or she got angry, someone got hurt either emotionally or physically. So Sam may have grown up with a fear of anger. Deep down in his unconscious he may be afraid of the consequences of his anger so he never lets it out.

But anger, along with other natural emotions, has to have an outlet. For a migraine sufferer this outlet may be a migraine. An ulcerative colitis sufferer may experience a colitis attack, but Sam has inherited a predisposition to psoriasis so for him the anger could be expressed through his skin in the form of psoriasis.

Psychotherapists probe the unconscious in search of these buried emotional clues. Writing in the book: *Who Can I talk to?*, published by Hodder and Stoughton, authors Judy Cooper and Jenny Lewis explain: 'Psychotherapy looks at a person's external and internal worlds. Our external worlds are our day-to-day activities as well as the events that occur in our lives and how we react to them. Our internal worlds are made up of memories, thoughts, dreams and fantasies that we are aware of as well as the desires, fears and fantasies that we are not conscious of. It is getting to know and understanding this internal world that is the art of psychotherapy. Skilfully done, it can unlock many doors for the patient and help to promote a positive and fulfilling lifestyle. Obviously, it is not a hit-and-miss affair. There are several techniques and intricate skills that the psychotherapist learns over many years.'

One of these techniques is the use of dreams. Again Cooper and Lewis explain: 'Psychoanalysis assumes that dreams have psychological meaning which can be arrived at by interpretation. In a dream state, a person is open to moods and feelings that are blocked or overshadowed while awake. By using dreams the therapist is able to unveil and clarify feelings and emotional patterns that are hidden from the patient.'

Even though dreams can seem very odd, there is actually not a great deal of difference between them and waking experiences. The main difference is in the language that is used. During consciousness we communicate in words, but during sleep we communicate in visual images. These visual images often have a symbolic meaning and it is interpreting these symbols and understanding what they mean that is the domain of the therapist.

Interpreting dreams can hold the key to the patient's unconscious fears as well as desires.

'When people start therapy, they are often unaware of having any dreams. But research tells us that people dream all the time. So it really is a question of learning to remember dreaming and the dream,' say Cooper and Lewis. Patients are apparently encouraged to keep pencil and paper or a tape recorder by their beds and to record whatever they remember when they wake up. It is not just the circumstances or situations in the dream that the therapist wants documented, but also the feelings that the dreams aroused. Most people apparently get into it quite quickly. *Who Can I talk to?* details all the major talking therapies available, describing what they are and whom they help. It is available from most book shops.

Coming face to face with unexpressed feelings can in itself discharge pent-up emotions. Learning why you hold on to patterns of behaviour, like, for example, not showing your anger, can take the restraint away to the extent that you can choose to carry on the way you are, or modify your behaviour. If, for example, Sam is no longer afraid of losing his temper because he is confident that he will never behave like the person who frightened him in his childhood, he may suddenly find that he doesn't shrink so much from confrontation. This may enable him to handle those kinds of situations more to his own satisfaction.

Obviously, this treatment takes time. Trust builds gradually in a relationship and this is true of psychotherapy too. Patients can be in treatment for many years but increasingly people can use it to good effect with short-term treatment lasting for a year or even less.

· *Counselling* ·

A counsellor's job is to look at the here and now and examine current patterns of behaviour. He or she will encourage you to talk freely without fear of being judged or criticised in any way. But the counsellor is also trained to try and relate current feelings and behaviour to things that have happened in the past. He or she will delve a little into childhood and family background to try and get a clearer picture of you as a person. The counsellor will, from time to time, reflect back what you have said to try to untangle the web of feelings and emotions engendered by a particular situation. Over a period of time, this kind of examination of why you do the things you do can help you to see yourself in a new light and help you to understand more about your feelings and motivations.

What counselling can also do is to help rid you of some of your emotional ghosts. Let's look, again, at Sam's unexpressed anger. During counselling the counsellor may have picked up that Sam has difficulty in expressing anger. Talking about it generally may lead Sam to recount the story of his outing with Jane. He will be encouraged to express his feelings about what took place. To this stranger with whom he has no relationship outside the counselling room he may be able to say how foolish and hurt he felt. He may be able to say how ashamed of himself he is at not having been able to handle the situation in a positive way. It may be the first time that Sam has ever been able to talk about the incident with anybody, let alone someone who is going to be sympathetic to him. This in itself may discharge some of the pent-up feelings of distress.

Then, with the counsellor's help, Sam may start to look at what happened when he was a child to see if there is a link there with his current behaviour. Sam may remember that when he was young, the family feared his father's temper because he shouted loudly, said unkind things which made his mother cry and threaten to leave and he and his sister were terrified. So for Sam anger may have become associated with fear, so now as an adult he recoils from it. Or Sam may resemble his father in many ways and unconsciously he may be afraid that he is like his father in this way too. He may be afraid that if he allows himself to feel angry, he will be angry and shout and terrify people like his father did.

Obviously, there are many permutations on the theme of Sam's problems with expressing anger, but the point is that when Sam is able to understand why anger is such a difficult issue for him, he may find that he is able to recognise when he is angry without being afraid of his anger. He may even be able to tell the person, 'You have made me angry because. . .' instead of bottling it up. So Sam can stop fearing his anger or worrying that he will behave like his father and instead start feeling more confident and happier about himself. And this may be reflected in the clearing of his psoriasis or, at least, an improvement in the condition.

It doesn't always work, of course, but it often does. These kinds of talking treatments are good at helping you to dispose of unwanted and destructive emotional baggage. They are also very useful in current emotional situations. If you are going through a bad patch or unhappy period of your life, talking to a counsellor can help you to express your anger and hurt and, in so doing, ease the pain.

The point to remember is that counselling is not supposed to be a destructive process – quite the contrary. The aim of peeling back the layers and helping you to know more about yourself is that it should strengthen you, give you more personal power and enable you to feel good about yourself.

· *Cognitive Therapy* ·

Cognitive therapy treats depression in a fairly pragmatic way. The theory is that people become depressed because they have a bad picture or low opinion of themselves. They may also have a pessimistic view of the outside world and feel that the future holds very little for them. They may be 'touchy', misinterpreting personal experiences so that things are seen in a negative way. For instance, they may be overly sensitive to casual remarks that are not intended to wound. This can easily happen in the case of psoriasis. The therapy aims to replace negative thinking with a more positive attitude to life.

Cognitive therapy is much more active than counselling or psychotherapy and the form it takes is often tailored to the individual client. Therapists believe that viewing oneself in a negative way is caused by irrational thought patterns that have become part of the person and the idea is to replace this irrational way of thinking with a more positive view.

Patients may be given homework like writing or drawing about personal experiences or other tasks that are agreed in the session by the client. Cognitive therapy is an off-shoot of behavioural therapy and is usually short-term.

· *Person-centered Psychotherapy* ·

This therapy was founded by an American psychologist called Dr. Carl Rogers. Person-centred therapists believe that, given the right conditions, everyone can achieve self-fulfilment and happiness.

One of the necessary conditions is what therapists call 'unconditional positive regard' from therapist to client. This basically means that the client receives from the therapist a feeling that he (or she) is an okay person regardless of who he is, what he looks like and what he or she has done. There are no judgements. Empathy is also considered to be essential for the client to be able to change his perspective of himself. This means that the therapist should understand who the client is, what he is feeling, what is his experience and its meaning and what he is trying to convey. The therapist is also required to be open and in touch with his or her own feelings and responses.

The idea is that once people become more in touch with who they are and what they really want, they can start to develop in their own way. Once people are put more in touch with themselves and start to understand what they want as opposed to what other people want of them, they can start to realise some of their own dreams and desires.

The therapist has no special interest in the client behaving in any particular way or being any particular kind of person. So the client can explore his or her own emotions and desires without any pressure or direction to be something or someone that family or friends may find acceptable. He is accepted for who he is at the time. This freedom of self-expression in an atmosphere of acceptance and confidentiality is believed to allow the patient to get to know himself and become the person he wants to be.

9

DOCTORS, CLINICS AND HOSPITALS

Treatment for psoriasis usually takes place in the doctor's surgery. Unless the condition is particularly severe or is not responding to treatment, your GP should be able to help you to bring your psoriasis under control. However, there are times when patients' needs are better met in out-patient clinics in hospitals. When the psoriasis is severe, as in erythrodermic or generalised pustular psoriasis and the patient is very ill, in-patient treatment is essential. But there are other reasons why people may be admitted for in-patient treatment. So let's have a look at all three situations and see what each has to offer.

· *The Surgery* ·

Psoriasis is a very individual illness, not only in the way it affects each person but in individual patients' perception of the severity of their condition and what they expect from treatment. If you speak to any nurse, doctor or specialist used to treating psoriatic patients, they will tell you that one patient's idea of bad psoriasis is a couple of patches while another will have lesions on various parts of their body and believe that their condition is mild.

Some patients will feel that their medication is working if it manages to clear just one area of their body, while others have a much higher expectation of their treatment.

Doctors and nurses treating psoriasis tend to feel that they should take their cue from the patient. So in many ways the ball is in your court.

This being the case, try to clarify in your own mind what you want from the treatment. Do this before you go to see the doctor. And be realistic! Maybe you have quite a wide coverage of psoriasis and would like to clear the lot. Are you prepared to devote time to the treatment? Or would you be better off concentrating on clearing the most significant areas first and worrying about the rest at another time?

One point you may like to consider is that success breeds success and failure breeds failure. If you set yourself a goal you can achieve without too much hassle, you will probably succeed and this will give you the optimism and confidence to tackle the next objective with a large degree of positivity. If you give yourself a very difficult target that you cannot possibly achieve without disrupting your entire life and perhaps not even then, the chances are that you will fail. You may achieve absolutely nothing and be left with an overwhelming feeling of hopelessness about your psoriasis. In other words, don't give yourself a hard time!

So decide what you want from the treatment and maybe write it down. Think about what matters to you most. Are there particular places on your body that you find difficult to treat? Which are the areas that bother you? Do you find the condition restrictive or disabling? What does it stop you from doing? What can you live with? What do you want to change?

The next step is to gather as much information about your psoriasis as you possibly can. When did it start? Are there particular times when it is bad? Have you had any adverse reactions from any treatments you have tried in the past? Have any been good? Are there any triggers you've noticed? These are just a few questions to set the ball rolling. Try to get as clear a picture of your psoriasis as you can.

If your psoriasis fluctuates quite regularly it may be worth keeping a diary to see if you can identify any patterns. Some people find that their condition gets bad at exam times. Stress triggers psoriasis for many people. However, there are some who are fine during stressful times, but when it is all over, psoriasis appears. Some people are helped by sunlight while others find that ultra-violet light exacerbates their condition. The more you know about your condition, the more likely you are to be able to find the most appropriate treatment to achieve your particular goal.

You may need to book a double appointment with the doctor. Just tell the receptionist that you will need a longer than normal time with the doctor and to book you a double slot.

In addition to examining you, the GP should listen to what you have to say and ask what you want from the treatment. Together with your views and his or her own perception of the severity of your psoriasis, the doctor should evaluate the situation and discuss possible treatments with you.

Between the two of you, you may decide that no other treatment is appropriate at this time. Talking to your doctor may be sufficient to establish in your mind that just using the emollients is as much as you need to do. Maybe it will encourage you to use the moisturisers more regularly! Or the doctor may feel that other topical treatment is required.

If this is the case the doctor should explain to you:

- What the treatment is.
- How you should apply it and how often.
- What you can expect it to achieve.
- What the side effects are.

And you should write this down. When you are sitting in the doctor's surgery you may think you understand everything and will remember it all, but once you've left, your mind goes blank. Writing it down on paper, even in note form, is a good memory aid.

The doctor may want to refer you to a consultant dermatologist or skin clinic. There may be a variety of reasons for this. Some of them are:

- If diagnosis is complicated and the doctor feels that it needs a more expert opinion.
- If you need to increase the amount of topical steroids you are taking.
- If you need systemic (tablet) treatment.
- If the doctor feels that you need help with learning to use and apply the topical treatments.
- If you need treatment that is only available in a hospital setting, like PUVA, for instance.
- If the condition is not responding to good topical treatment which is being applied properly and as often as prescribed. (You usually have to give the treatment a good three months before deciding that it is not producing the results required.)
- If you have a very severe form of the condition like erythrodermic or generalised pustular psoriasis, which needs instant in-patient treatment.

Whether or not you are referred to a dermatologist may also depend on how much knowledge your doctor has about skin complaints. Some GPs are very keen and clued up about many of the new treatments available and will be confident about managing most of their psoriasis patients themselves. Other doctors may have a special interest in other conditions like, for instance, diabetes or cardiology, and not be so up-to-date on what is happening in the world of dermatology. So at what stage you may be referred to a specialist can vary from doctor to doctor.

A very important factor to notice in your consultation with your doctor is his or her attitude to psoriasis. Many GPs understand the situation with psoriasis and are well aware of what their patients are going through. They know that there is as yet no cure but they have the patience and the interest to ensure that their patients get the help available to enable them to keep their condition under control.

Sadly, there are still some doctors who believe that because there is no cure for psoriasis and because it is such a frustrating illness to treat, there is nothing they can do for you. This is absolutely untrue. If you find that your doctor has this attitude, ask to be referred to a specialist. Every patient is entitled to a second opinion on his or her condition and seeing a dermatologist is getting a second opinion. Your doctor should not deny you this.

In the final analysis, if you are not getting the help you need from your GP, you can always move to another one.

· *Changing Doctors* ·

It is normally very easy to change doctors; what you first have to do is to find another one to take you on. Do a bit of research. See what other practices have to offer. Do any of the doctors have a special interest in skin conditions? If there is a surgery that you know is good or have heard good things about on the grapevine, make an appointment with one of the senior doctors. Tell him or her that you have psoriasis and to what extent you would like to clear it. Ask what kind of treatments he or she would consider using to help you to keep it under control.

Don't worry about asking these kinds of questions. People are often very worried about asking too many questions and wasting the doctor's time. Bear in mind that a doctor who is patient with your questioning is also likely to be patient and understanding of your psoriasis. Some doctors have a problem with patients with chronic illnesses like psoriasis. They get very frustrated with conditions they cannot cure. Others have a more realistic understanding of the problem.

Assuming you have found a doctor that you want to move to, first make sure that the practice is willing to take you on. If they are, you may now have to write to your current doctor and tell him that you are moving and where you are moving to. This is so that your medical records are sent on to the new practice. You don't have to give the outgoing doctor any reasons for your move. You will then need to wait a couple of weeks for your medical records to reach their new destination – and that's it.

If you would like any more information on changing doctors you can ring the Regional Health Information Service on 0800 665544. This is a national number which you ring and are automatically put through to your region. If you want to know how to make a comment or complaint about the health service, operators on this line can usually point you in the right direction to get help.

· *Day Care Clinics* ·

One of the most significant modern innovations in psoriatic care has been the development of day-care programmes in hospitals. Whereas previously people would have been admitted to hospital to have their tar baths, tar applications and dithranol treatments, now many hospitals are able to offer this on a day-care basis. Patients attend the dermatology unit, usually for a couple of hours a day. Some will attend every day which of course speeds up treatment, but not everybody can afford that amount of time and may come two or three times a week which means that the condition is likely to take longer to clear.

Treatments given on a day-care basis are quite varied. Some patients will receive short contact dithranol treatment following UVB therapy. This is known as the modified Ingrams regimen. Very resistant types of psoriasis may be treated with PUVA therapy followed by short contact dithranol.

PUVA is a combination of long-wave ultra-violet A (UVA) and a photosensitising agent called psoralens (P). Psoralens can be taken by mouth in tablet form or applied to the skin as either paint/emulsion or added to water (Bath PUVA). Ultra-violet light treatment is always given prior to the application of topical treatments.

The treatment does not have to be complex to qualify for the day-care programmes. There are various reasons why people come to hospital for treatment. Sometimes patients cannot reach the parts of the body that need treating and may not necessarily have someone who can help them. Or they may not be able to stand the mess, the staining and the smell at home, particularly if a large area of the body needs treating.

Ultra-violet treatment needs to be carried out in hospital. The machines have to be properly calibrated and it is important that trained staff measure the dose of UV that their patients are receiving.

Some patients may come just for the tar applications and the baths. Others will come for their scalps to be treated. People with thick scalp psoriasis can have a problem treating it themselves. A trained nurse can apply the preparations more efficiently and therefore render the treatment more effective.

The day-care clinics are nurse-led. Specially trained dermatology nurses assess the patient's condition and manage all their treatments and care while they are going through the programme. Of course, there are protocols and guidelines that the nurses have to follow and if a problem arises they can refer to a dermatologist for a second opinion.

The day-care programmes are able to overcome some of the problems of contemporary medical care. Now that hospital beds are at a premium, these clinics bridge the gap between in-patient treatment and leaving patients to treat the condition on their own.

Apart from the application of creams and ultra-violet therapy, day-care clinics also offer an educational programme. Lynette Stone, a dermatology nurse at St. John's Institute of Dermatology and Chair of the British Dermatological Nursing Group, explains: 'One of the major issues with anyone with psoriasis is that they are very self-conscious about they way they look. They also may well not understand much about the condition.

'A huge element of any day-care programme, as far as the nursing input is concerned, is in providing an education for patients so that they know how to do their treatment properly. They also learn about their condition and we can work out some plan with them that they can carry out at home to help them keep the condition under control.' This will include an action plan that patients can adopt during the times when the psoriasis flares up. Bringing the condition quickly under control is the goal. But how this is achieved varies widely from person to person.

All psoriasis patients need to keep their skin moisturised through the use of simple emollients, but some people may also need a course of ultra-violet treatment without psoralen to keep their condition under control. Other patients might need topical ointments for psoriasis; some may respond best to PUVA treatment and some will need to be on drugs like Cyclosporin or the retinoids. They all have the same diagnosis of psoriasis but they each need a different therapy to get it under control. And finding out which is best for you helps you to tackle the flare-up with confidence and can take some of the stress out of the situation. So part of the education is keeping patients in touch with all the developments and treatments.

'Doing the treatments can take a long time,' says Lynette Stone, 'and one of the things we're finding now is that because of the pressure on beds we have patients referred whom we would not have expected, because such large areas of their body are affected. It can sometimes take the nurses an hour or more just to apply the treatment.

'Since the nurses spend such a long time with patients actually doing the treatment, there is plenty of opportunity for them to chat about any problems or issues in a more relaxed way. So they can give information or try to sort out problems. Many patients may need quite a lot of emotional or psychological support to help them cope with their condition. The nurses can do this while applying the treatment, so it's done in a very informal setting.'

The length of day-care treatment varies from person to person, depending on how bad the condition is and how many days in a week the patient attends, but three weeks is the average. It can depend on what the patient wants out of the treatment. Clearing up designated patches on the body is going to take less time than achieving total clearance, which is the preferred goal of some patients.

There is a move towards developing the role of specially trained dermatology nurses. An option currently being examined is the development of the post of a dermatology community liaison nurse who would be able to talk to and advise patients in situations that do not require a doctor.

· *In-Patient Treatment* ·

People are admitted to hospital as in-patients for a variety of reasons. They may be erythrodermic or have acute pustular psoriasis and be severely ill. Or so much of their body may be affected that they cannot be looked after on a day-care basis. Some patients may not be able to manage the travelling or they may be elderly and frail. Women whose psoriasis flares up during pregnancy may be treated on an in-patient basis.

Any one of these situations can cause a patient to be admitted into hospital care. However, the most common reason for admission is when the patient has an extensive coverage of psoriasis which makes him or her generally unwell. When psoriasis dominates large areas of the skin, patients are likely to experience problems that require expert handling. They may have a problem with temperature control. They may be losing body heat. Their fluid balance may be badly affected. They are likely to be at risk of secondary infection. They hurt. They feel dreadful and if their general condition isn't properly treated they can become very ill.

People who are erythrodermic or have generalised pustular psoriasis may need special airbeds to be nursed on so that their skin doesn't get more damaged. A patient who is likely to lose a great deal of skin every time he or she moves needs extremely sensitive, considered and specialised nursing. The fluctuating temperature will need to be monitored and the fluid intake kept up.

As with day-care, the average time spent in hospital for most people with psoriasis is three weeks. Patients with the severe forms of the condition may need to stay in for three to four months. Those who have particularly unstable psoriasis may find it takes several weeks, if not months, to get the condition to settle down.

However, patients are not always referred for in-patient treatment because of the severity of their psoriasis. Occasionally it is to relieve a domestic situation. There may be all kinds of pressures within a marriage but sometimes the psoriasis is the main focus. In such a case the objective would be to offer the person in-patient treatment to gain control of the illness by intensive topical treatments. At the same time support, counselling and education are offered to the patient and partner to ease the situation and help them to plan how to cope with possible further outbreaks of psoriasis.

'You can't look at it as just treating the skin,' says Lynette Stone. 'You've got to look at the whole family and the dynamics of the situation.'

Remission time for psoriasis varies, regardless of whether people are treated on a day-care or in-patient basis. Some patients will be clear for years. Others return regularly every year for three weeks of treatment. It may seem like a large investment in time, but some people opt for this because it enables them to keep their condition under control and live their lives the rest of the time as they want to, without placing an extra strain on their families.

Patients whose psoriasis is going through an unstable phase may find that their remission time is very short. They may be clear when they leave hospital but maintaining the remission can be difficult during the unstable period.

Finally, there are patients who do not keep up the treatments prescribed when they get home so their remission time can also be very short.

· *The Singing Detective* ·

This play by Dennis Potter, which was first broadcast on BBC Television in 1986, did a great deal to bring psoriasis into the public domain. The hospital setting in which much of the action takes place certainly struck a familiar chord with many psoriasis sufferers who had themselves spent many weeks of many years in the general wards of hospitals. The play had a big impact on viewers, so much so that even now it can be used as a quick way of telling people what psoriasis is. Ever experienced this bit of dialogue?

'I suffer from psoriasis'.

'What's that?'

'*The Singing Detective?*'

'Oh *that!*'

Potter himself suffered from severe psoriasis and psoriatic arthritis and through his main character, Philip Marlow, was able very empathetically to paint a graphic picture of the condition.

Philip Marlow is a detective story writer who is in hospital with psoriasis and psoriatic arthritis. He is covered from head to foot with lesions and the arthritis is so bad that he cannot move. He is a picture of misery lying in a prison of pain unable even to move from his bed to get a packet of cigarettes which the nurses have placed on top of his locker and out of his reach.

Marlow's books are out of print and his marriage is on the rocks. In the first part of the play he lies there seething with anger but defenceless and dependent on hospital staff who are not particularly sensitive either to his condition or his predicament. Potter describes it as such:

'*Marlow is wearing only a tiny loincloth – normal practice when seeing a dermatology consultant – exposing his hideously disfigured skin to clinical gaze.*

'*He is helplessly flat on his back, laid out like a corpse, on top of the bed clothes, on a paper sheet already soaked with grease.*'

Marlow's skin is inflamed, his temperature is high and he is on the verge of hallucinating. He is very ill. The consultant asks him questions which he starts to answer but is ignored. The doctors seem to be much more interested in exchanging views with each other than in considering anything their patient has to say. Fortunately, this kind of attitude is becoming far rarer in modern medicine, but those of us who have been made to feel incidental to our own illnesses may enjoy Potter's unique handling of the situation.

The consultant speaks to Marlow:

There's another drug which might help you. Mr–ah– How do you feel about trying one of the new retinoids, mmm?

Absolute silence. Marlow does not attempt to speak, not this time. The pause lengthens, comically. They all look at each other. The consultant leans in to speak again, as though to a retarded child.

Do-you-understand-the-question?

Marlow: No I don't think so.

Consultant: I am asking if you'd–

Marlow: (cutting in) I don't understand because I seem to have regressed into the helpless and pathetic condition of total dependency. Of the kind normally associated with infancy.

Astonishment. The consultant, who was leaning in, straightens like a shot.

Visiting Doctor: (Astounded) What's he say?' But Marlow, who can scarcely lift his head, and who is burning up, gives them the full blast, and not at all calm.

Marlow: The last time I experienced anything remotely like this was in my bloody pram! Being drooled over by slobbering cretins –

Sister Malone: Mr Marlow –!

Marlow: – who turned out to be escapees from the local loony bin. They thought they were doctors and nurses.

In the event the consultant laughs.

It is an intricate plot which combines the story of Marlow's childhood, his fantasy world in which he is The Singing Detective and his progress in the ward during the months in hospital.

His childhood is a traumatic one. He sees his mother making love to a school friend's father. He is terrorised by a particularly sadistic teacher whose memory still haunts him. He has to leave his home and his father to live in London during which time his first psoriatic patch appears. And soon after this his mother dies.

In sharp contrast to his crippled and almost lifeless self, his other persona, The Singing Detective, is highly mobile and capable and is out and about in bars and river banks, venues very different from hospital wards, solving international crime.

In hospital Marlow is receiving both drug and topical treatments but, in addition, he is taken regularly in his wheelchair to see Dr. Gibbon, the psychotherapist. Although Marlow is not particularly sympathetic to Dr. Gibbon, one gets the impression that the sessions help to trigger the trips down Memory Lane. Bit by bit as the childhood story unfurls both in the consulting room and in flashback scenes, Gibbon notices that Marlow is able to move more easily. First he is able to move his neck more flexibly. Then he is able to type a little and eventually he is able to stand up unaided.

At the end Marlow the writer, who has also shed his lesions, is visited in his hospital bed by Marlow, The Singing Detective who says: *'Only one of us is going to walk out of here. Sweeter than the roses.'*

Marlow walks out of hospital into the outside world, leaning on his wife for support.

The Singing Detective, by Dennis Potter is published in paperback by Faber and Faber priced £7.99. It is immensely readable.

· *Patch Tests* ·

These are done to discover if you are allergic to any substance that comes in contact with your skin. They are usually carried out in the dermatology clinic. The dermatologist will ask for details of your skin problems and the kind of materials you handle at work or use regularly at home or in the course of a hobby or social activity. He or she will also examine your skin and ask about substances that you could be sensitive to (such as nickel, found in rings and other jewellery).

A diluted version of each possible allergen is then put on different areas of a piece of filter paper which is then applied to an unaffected area of your body usually your back. The paper is stuck on with some adhesive tape and left in place for 48 hours. The patch is then removed and the skin is examined. You may then be asked to return 48 hours after that when the skin is examined again. It is very important to return for this check. If the skin is itchy, red and swollen in some places, the dermatologist will check what was on that particular area or areas of filter paper to determine what it is you are allergic to.

You can then try to avoid the substances that cause the problem. Although patch testing sounds simple, getting the solutions right is quite a complex business and you shouldn't try to do it yourself. It really is a specialist's job!

· *Sheila* ·

Sheila has had psoriasis for 27 years. It occurred after a traumatic incident when her 18-month-old daughter fell down an open stairway. The child fell on to her face and the teeth that she had cut at 18 months went back into the gum and the gum caved in. Her face was covered in blood. Two weeks after that Sheila noticed her first psoriatic patch on her elbow. She had never heard of psoriasis until then.

I went to the doctor for something else and she saw the patch on my elbow and told me that it was psoriasis. She gave me some steroid cream to put on and told me to forget about it. But it gradually got worse. It spread all over and went on to my legs, hands, feet and then on to my body.

After two or three years I was referred to a specialist who admitted me into hospital for the first time. I was there for about three weeks. I had a thick tar paste applied all over my body. I was more or less covered from head to foot. It was left on all day and all night and every day new tar was put on top of the old tar. I was allowed to have two baths a week.

At the end of the three weeks I was clear but I only stayed clear for three weeks. At the time I said that I would never go into hospital again because it wasn't worth it, but in fact my psoriasis gets so bad that I go in every year and have done for the last 20 years. And I still have the same treatment.

On average I'm in for a month each year. It was very difficult when the children were small because I'd have to get my parents to move into my house and help my husband to look after them. Looking back on it now I wonder how I coped, but you do. I had no choice. I had tried all the creams the doctor had given me to no avail and I had to get some relief. As it happens, the specialist wasn't happy about the fact that I had been prescribed all those steroid creams.

I've always taken the view that when I go into hospital I've got to switch off. There's no point going in if you're going to start worrying about the children, the home and everything else. They say it is a stress-related complaint and if you worry about home you are not going to get better in hospital.

When I first come out of hospital I always continue the tar treatment at home. It is very messy. But if we're going on holiday I want to be nice and clear so I put up with it. It is difficult to do at home but because I don't go out to work, I persevere. I put the tar on in the morning when I get up and leave it on for about three hours. And then I do it again perhaps at night when I am sitting and watching television. Occasionally I go to bed with tar and all sorts of bandages on, but I try not to do that because I get so hot anyway and it's not fair on my husband. My skin is usually clear for a month after I come out of hospital.

We've got a son who lives in Corfu and obviously I like to go and see him. We always go late in the season because I am worse in hot weather. My skin is bad in the sun. But this year for the first time my skin was fine. I used Factor 30. We didn't do a lot of sunbathing because I can't do that now. But I was sitting on the beach playing with my grandchildren. I made sure that I sat under an umbrella and my skin was perfect. It hasn't been like that in the past. By the second week in the holiday my skin is usually bad, so while everybody else is in shorts and bikinis I am covered up and feeling hot and miserable.

I only wear short sleeves when I come out of hospital and my skin is clear. When my skin is bad on my hands I don't want to go out. If I can cover up the psoriasis it's okay. But if I can see it I know that other people can see it and then I won't go out, particularly if we are going for a meal. I feel so awful about it and I feel that it is off-putting for other people, even though my friends and family say it doesn't bother them.

I find the worst part of psoriasis is the way you look and feel. You don't feel clean. Even though you're covered up you know that it's all there underneath.

The summer of 1995 was a nightmare in hospital. I was in there in August. A lot of the time the temperature was in the 80's. We've got a new purpose-built ward at Clatterbridge for dermatology, but there is no air conditioning. I had tar all over my body and bandages over that and I was wearing gloves. It was unbearable.

Over the years I've got to know the nurses at the hospital and many of the other patients as well. There's usually someone I know when I go in, which is nice. I've made a lot of friends through the psoriasis ward and I keep in touch with some of them.

It would be awful if they took the ward away from us. I don't know what we'd do, because what we'd have then would be a couple of beds in either a medical or a surgical ward and that would be horrendous. We feel so awful. When you're in a dermatology ward, some people may have eczema or leg ulcers, but everybody is in the same boat. They know what it is all about. So you relax. You don't worry about your complaint.

If you went into a medical or surgical ward it would be completely different. Lots of people don't know what psoriasis is. They'd shun you because they'd think you'd got something catching.

A psoriasis patient whom I know went in to have her appendix out and the other women in her bay said that she shouldn't be in that ward. They wanted her moved. They thought she had something catching. You can't relax in those circumstances.

Knowing that if the psoriasis gets really bad I can go into hospital is very important to me. No matter how hard I try I cannot get rid of it myself. I need the rest I get in hospital. I need to get a breather from the psoriasis and all the problems it causes. I also know that when I come out of hospital my skin will be clear. I will be able to wear what I like and go where I like. And even though it only lasts for a month I look forward to it all year.

· *Bill* ·

Bill has had psoriasis for over 50 years. He has had psoriatic arthritis for much of that time. Both the rash and the arthritis have been constant companions for most of his life and Bill has been an in-patient in hospital between 20 and 25 times. However, Bill has had a successful career and led an active life. He says he has been extremely fortunate in having a very tolerant and supportive wife. They have been married for 48 years. Here Bill gives an account of how the psoriasis first started and he also describes in-patient dithranol treatment as he experienced it in the past and as he receives it now. Bill is in his mid-seventies.

I was a 19-year-old service man, serving with the ground staff of the Royal Air Force in Iraq and the Persian Gulf, when I first developed psoriasis. I suppose I was under a certain amount of stress. In common with thousands of others, I had spent many weeks in crowded conditions in troopships, with the ever-present threat of submarine attacks. The climate in the Persian Gulf, in those days before any sort of air-conditioning, was quite rigorous. With the temperature round about 100 degrees F, I managed to fall ill with pneumonia, which put me in hospital for about three months. It was around about this time when I first saw signs of psoriasis.

The first thing I noticed was a thickening of the toe nails and then a very large patch of dry skin appeared on my thigh. It wasn't diagnosed as psoriasis until two or three years later.

After the end of the War I trained as an accountant. One of the principals I was working closely with died under rather unfortunate circumstances. My skin had always been troublesome since my return to the UK, but it started to get a lot worse and then the psoriatic arthritis appeared. In fact the arthritis was a much greater problem than the rash.

It started off in my hands and then it became pretty widespread. Every joint you could think of was affected and eventually I was flat out in hospital for quite a long time. In those days they used to give gold injections for arthritis. I didn't experience a great deal of comfort from that.

I go into hospital quite regularly. It gets to a point when the psoriasis becomes very wearing. I have a sympathetic consultant who takes me into hospital. I spend about three weeks there and I come out very much more comfortable.

Over the years I have had all manner of treatments. I have had all the drugs you can think of and PUVA treatment, but I find that the only things that really help are the topical treatments like dithranol. The only trouble is that as I get older I become less tolerant of it. I used to be able to take quite strong doses but nowadays unless I have a fairly weak strength it does affect me quite badly. So then they have to start treating me for the burns.

It was a strain when I was younger. I used to work in the City of London and I found that almost every year I took time out to go into hospital. What I normally did was to take a couple of weeks of my annual holiday to go into hospital so that it did not affect my work quite so much. Sometimes it would flare up and I'd have an unpleasant month or so and then it would die down again and not be too bad.

The rash is in large patches on my body. For a long time the actual trunk wasn't affected, but I've always had it on my arms, legs, back and scalp. It is very itchy and it can get painful too. At home I am very lucky. I have an extremely tolerant wife.

Fortunately until just recently I could cover it up. People couldn't see it. They didn't know that I was a mess under my clothing. But it meant I couldn't go swimming which I always used to enjoy. The doctors tell you 'of course you can go swimming', but if people like us were to go into a swimming bath everyone else would get out. We know it is not contagious but the general public doesn't know that. It's natural. I am sure I'd be exactly the same myself. Recently the psoriasis has come on to my hands.

I have very little treatment now for the arthritis. I am affected in the hands, feet and neck at the moment. I can get around. I use a stick but I'm mobile.

I find that nowadays when I go into hospital I know quite a number of the staff. They seem like old friends. It is not nearly as bad when you're in as the contemplation of going in.

In hospital I am put on dithranol treatment. It's a much higher potency than the one that you use at home and they have to monitor it very carefully. I start the day with a bath in tar solution. It's an emollient with a tar base to soften up the skin. Then they put the dithranol pastes on in varying degrees of strength. They start off with a very low potency one and then they build it up. In the past I used to be able to take quite a strong one. Nowadays I can't do that.

The old system was that you were then put into a stockinet. And you kept that on for 24 hours when you took it off, had your bath and started the whole procedure again. Sometimes they would ring the changes. You would have the stockinet put on for three days and then for the next two days they would wrap you up in polythene.

This particular system has changed. They do the dithranol treatment in the same way, but they have found that the polythene and stockinet is not really necessary so they don't do that any more. Nowadays they put a liberal coating of talcum powder all over you after you have had the dithranol applied. This is to stop the dithranol spreading to unaffected parts and burning. And you just sit around in your pyjamas.

So you have the bath in the morning, have the dithranol applied and then after about 12 hours they top up the dithranol and that stays on until the next morning when you have the tar bath. It is still a 24-hour process. In my case this goes on for anything from two to three weeks.

When I am out of hospital I use the short contact dithrocream or a steroid cream and I can usually keep my skin fairly controlled for about five or six months before it becomes uncomfortable again.

I find the psoriasis worse than the arthritis. Arthritis is difficult and painful but you can get used to the pain of arthritis. Psoriasis can become extremely uncomfortable. It is sometimes very difficult to find a way of sitting or even standing without it being painful.

Socially it can be embarrassing but I have a lot of very good friends and they accept it. It's when you're amongst strangers that it is difficult. But I'm pretty thick-skinned about it nowadays.

When my skin is scaling and my wife and I go away to a hotel we take a dustpan and brush with us. It can be embarrassing.

It has affected my life to the extent that there are quite a number of things I would like to have done. For instance on holiday there is no way I can wear shorts and short-sleeved shirts. I do enjoy going to warmish places but it means that I am always in long trousers and long sleeves. It can feel a bit strange sometimes if everyone else is floating around in bikinis and shorts.

10

CHILDREN AND TEENAGERS

Psoriasis often makes its first appearance in childhood. Puberty is a very common time for it to start, particularly with girls. The initial trigger is often stress caused by exams or a change of school or upheaval in the home environment.

Psoriasis can be as isolating for children as it is for adults. But it doesn't have to be. Learning to handle the condition in childhood socially and physically can stand the patient in very good stead in later life. If you discover as a child that you can be successful and popular despite what you look like, you are probably light years ahead of your peer group in terms of emotional maturity and inner stability.

The treatments for psoriasis in childhood are similar to those in adulthood and many of the social problems may also run along the same lines. Some children may go through a bad patch if they have to put up with a lot of teasing. Many will have problems handling activities like sport, swimming and the embarrassment of having to dress and undress in communal changing rooms.

One of the most valuable things you can do for a child with psoriasis is to tell him or her as much as you can about the condition. Children are extremely vulnerable to other people's ignorance, particularly to the ignorance of their friends' parents.

If your child has psoriasis, make sure that he knows that it is not catching and tell him to tell his friends. Give your child the words with which to fight back. If you are at all friendly with the parents of your child's friends, tell them about psoriasis, making sure that they know that it is not catching.

If your child feels loved and valued he will have an inner strength that will help to carry him through the teasing or unpleasantness. A child with psoriasis may feel messy and unlovable so you may need to counteract this with plenty of hugs and cuddles. You may be a naturally tactile family or you may not. If you are not, you may need to reconsider this in the light of the psoriasis. A child with psoriasis needs to get the unspoken message that, in spite of his skin and the messiness of his treatments, he is good to touch. He or she may need the physical reinforcement of love and affection to enable him to regard the skin condition as something that does not have to get in the way of a normal, happy life with good relationships.

Many adults feel relieved when a mysterious illness is diagnosed, sometimes even if the condition is a serious one. Children can be sensitive and imaginative but they often cannot put their thoughts into words. So it is not uncommon for children to feel that it is their fault that they have got a condition like psoriasis. They've done something wrong or there is something inferior about them. Having the condition explained can go a long way towards helping children to cope with it. Talk about psoriasis in an open way and encourage your child and other members of the family to do the same. This way if your child is teased he may think that there is something deficient about the taunter and convey this message in return which could bring the teasing to an abrupt end.

Encourage your child to do the things that other children do, even though at times it may be awkward or difficult. Staying with friends overnight, for instance, which is such an enjoyable part of childhood, can pose problems for a child with psoriasis. Try to find ways to help your child enjoy sleep-overs without worrying too much. Since he or she may not be able to do the moisturising that night, it may be worth paying special attention to the skin-care routine a few days earlier, if you know about the sleep-over in advance. A well moisturised skin is far less likely to be flaky.

Warn the host-parent of your child's condition, explaining, of course, that it is not catching. Let your son or daughter take his or her own sleeping bag, pillow and towel. Explain to the parent that your child may be embarrassed about undressing in front of anyone, including his friend, and that if he wants to sleep the night in his day-time clothes, he should be allowed to do so.

· *Home Life* ·

Children like to be the same as everybody else. It can sometimes be extremely difficult when you are trying to make a child with psoriasis feel very loved, to convey the message that he or she is no different from the other family members. So here are some pointers to consider:

● Don't make one law for him and another for the other children in the family. Treat them all the same even though you may feel especially protective of your child with psoriasis.

- Talk. Many people reach adult life unable to share their feelings with others. They have grown up with the impression that they have to keep their thoughts and feelings to themselves for fear of being thought weak and vulnerable. Having feelings is not being weak. It is being normal. And in one way or another we are all vulnerable. A child who has psoriasis may have some very negative feelings about his condition. If he can learn to share these feelings with family and friends, not only will it ease the burden of the condition, but he will become a much more open and emotionally confident person. And if stress is a trigger, talking can go a long way to alleviating stress which may in turn have a beneficial effect on the skin condition.

- Don't be over-protective. Let your child do the same things as his siblings and friends do unless, of course, the state of his skin at any particular time dictates otherwise. Try to promote the notion of joining in rather than opting out.

- Include siblings. A child with psoriasis can take up a lot of time in the skin-care routine. Obviously you may not be able to ask the other children to help you when it comes to putting on preparations like tar or dithranol, but see if they can be in the room while you're doing the treatments, so that they can join in the chat and feel part of the whole process. If you can make the treatment routine a time for being together and cosy it will put a very different complexion on the condition than if you give the impression that the treatment is a chore and something to be got out of the way.

- If your son or daughter has to go into hospital as an in-patient for treatment, talk about it. Explain why he is going in and, if you can, what is likely to happen. If he is very young, make sure that he knows that it is only for a short time and that he will soon be coming home.

- Get your child to take as much responsibility for his psoriasis as possible. As soon as he can learn to apply the emollients, let him do so. The more children can feel in charge of looking after their condition themselves, the more confidence they will have about doing different activities, visiting friends, sleeping-over and so on, and the less the psoriasis will rule their lives and yours.

· *School Life* ·

One of the most valuable allies your child can have is an informed and sympathetic teacher. So make a point of going to see the head teacher or your child's class or form teacher. You may need to do this every year as the teacher changes. Book an appointment for about 15 minutes and ask the teacher to try to make sure you won't be interrupted. This will avail you of his or her undivided attention and it will also give the teacher the impression that you take your child's skin condition seriously.

Explain the condition briefly. It is one that is caused by the skin renewing itself at a much faster rate than normal which is what produces the plaques and causes the skin to flake. *Ensure that the teacher knows that the condition is not catching* and strongly encourage him or her to share this information with the rest of the class. If the child's classmates can be told about psoriasis by the teacher, much of the teasing can be nipped in the bud.

If your child's psoriasis is itchy, explain this to the teacher and say that your child is not being disruptive and that telling him or her not to scratch is not going to help matters. Explain that the itchiness can be very stressful and that if the child could be allowed to leave the classroom to apply some emollient it may ease the situation. This does mean, of course, that you will need to remember to pack a small tube of emollient into your child's school bag.

A cool corner of the classroom, away from radiators is important for a child with psoriasis, particularly if the condition is itchy.

If your child has psoriasis on his hands, activities which include the use of some materials may aggravate the condition. Play dough, finger paints, sand and water play are examples. It may be that the child can get by with the application of emollient beforehand to act as a barrier, washing well after and re-applying the cream. For older children glues, paints, clay, chemicals, oils and detergents can pose problems. Cotton mittens or plastic gloves, emollients, washing or showering after the activity with time given for the re-application of creams may be all that is needed to enable the child to take part. However, in some cases the child will need to be excused a particular activity.

Soaps, washing-up liquids and paper towels can all irritate the skin. Provide your child with a soap-substitute, emollient and cotton towel.

As regards sport, although it is important for your child to join in as much as possible, there may be times when he may not be able to take part. If the skin is dry and splitting, your child may not be able to do gym or other sports that require stretching.

You may also need to discuss with the teacher the fact that your child may be reluctant to go swimming or join in sporting activities because of the embarrassment factor. Undressing in front of others if your skin is sore and flaky takes a lot of courage as does appearing in a bathing costume in that condition. If your child's teacher has not come across psoriasis before, he or she may not be aware of the psychological implications.

Your child's teacher may have come across children with eczema and feel that psoriasis is more or less the same. Although they are both skin conditions and may at times look similar, they are quite different.

The Psoriasis Association can provide literature for you to take to the school. They will also write to the school if you think that this would help you or your child.

· *Teenagers* ·

Psoriasis can often occur for the first time during the teenage years and if it is already there, it can get worse in times of stress like exams or going to college or leaving home for a job far away.

Treatments are much the same as for adults. But it can be difficult to manage some of the social pressures in adolescence particularly if the psoriasis is severe.

To psyche yourself into going out and meeting new people in pubs, clubs and discos when your skin is looking bad can take quite a bit of courage. Sunbathing on the beach with your friends could be embarrassing. But bear in mind that skin is not always at its best during the teenage years and many of your friends may be having a hard time with acne.

If you possibly can, put the nervousness or embarrassment to one side and go out and do what you want to do. If your friends are going to the beach, join in. And if the sun is good for your psoriasis, don't cover your skin completely. Let it see the sun – in moderation, of course. If you can disregard the embarrassment factor at this stage of your life (and goodness knows it's difficult) you are much more likely to be laid back about your skin as you get older. If you acquire the frame of mind that you are the same as everybody else and have an equal right to enjoy your life, you will probably do just that.

You can, of course, help the skin condition by regular moisturising. If you keep your skin well moisturised you will get rid of the scales. If it gets dry, not only will your skin flake but it may crack and it can also become itchy. Keep yourself fit by eating healthy food.

If you find that you get unduly stressed over exams, try and learn some form of relaxation. Meditation, self-hypnosis and relaxation tapes are available and some of them can make you feel very relaxed. Here are some other pointers:

Shopping for clothes can sometimes be a problem because of the communal dressing rooms. You can say to the assistant that you haven't got time to try the clothes on now, so would it be okay to pay for them, try them on at home, but return them and get your money back if they don't fit. Many shops will agree. If you know your size and can identify the shops that sell the clothes that you like and fit you well, you can possibly buy them off the shelf. Many people with psoriasis buy their clothes through mail order outlets.

Hairdressers can be insensitive to people with scalp psoriasis, but some are extremely helpful. Having a hairstyle that you like and that suits you can do an enormous amount to boost your confidence, so don't give up on hairdressers just because you've had a bad experience with one. If you want to save yourself a lot of embarrassment and hassle, telephone the hairdressers of your choice first. Tell them that you have psoriasis on your scalp and explain what it is and what it is not. And then ask them if this is going to be a problem for them. If they are at all vague or strange on the phone, give them a miss and move on to the next one on your list. Sooner or later you will find one who is both skilful and kind.

Alternatively, you may like to find a hairdresser who makes home visits. Many people who are housebound for various reasons have hairdressers who visit them. These are often trained and skilful people who prefer, perhaps because of their own commitments, to work in a freelance way in people's homes rather than in a salon setting.

Staying over may present problems if you are embarrassed about the state of your skin. Take your own sleeping bag, towel and pillow. If you possibly can, try to have a quick shower and moisturise your skin before going to bed. It will stop it from flaking the next morning. A quick way to moisturise your skin is to stand in the bath or shower while still wet, smooth some baby oil into your skin and then gently pat it dry. It is a lick-and-promise moisturising tip but it can be a useful thing to do if you're staying with friends and do not want to occupy the bathroom for too long. Be sure to rinse the bath or shower out properly afterwards to remove the oil.

Dating can be a worry, but do bear in mind that most people with psoriasis are married and have children and grandchildren. So, although your skin may bother you, by and large it doesn't seem to put other people off, particularly once they have got to know you.

If your psoriasis is on a part of your body that is visible, the problem is more in first impressions when meeting new people. If it is elsewhere on the body and you have always managed to cover up, the worry comes later. As the relationship becomes more physically intense, so does the dilemma about whether you should say anything or not.

Why not mention it early on when it looks as if the relationship is going to take off? How can you enjoy being with the other person in a relaxed way with something like this weighing on your mind? The fear of rejection haunts most people at various stages of their lives, but at few times more so than in adolescence. It is not exclusive to people with psoriasis. Most of us fear rejection and most of us find something to pin it on. We may be short, overweight, shy, find it difficult to make small-talk, and so on.

It may be easier to tell your friend what's on your mind rather than shuffling around and making excuses because you're afraid of the crunch. If you duck and dive too much you run the risk of setting up a chain of misunderstandings or causing the other person to wonder if you've 'gone funny'. It's much better just to come out with words to the effect of: 'I've got this skin condition called psoriasis. It's not catching and you probably haven't noticed it because I've kept it covered up. But the skin on my arms and legs looks awful. Do you still want to go out with me?'

Careers are worth considering at this stage since the type of work that you do can have a bearing on your psoriasis. If your skin condition is more than very mild, stressful or physically and emotionally demanding occupations such as those within the police force or the armed forces can aggravate the condition.

If you have psoriasis on your hands, it may be best to stay away from careers that are going to expose them to a lot of chemicals or even get them consistently wet. Hairdressing, for instance, may be a problem for someone with hand psoriasis. Engineering, where you would be working with oils and other types of grease, may also be difficult and nursing where you are in contact with irritants and are constantly washing your hands may make the psoriasis worse.

If you have psoriasis on your feet, careers in which you will be standing a lot of the time should be avoided.

· *Rob* ·

Rob is 21 years old. He has had psoriasis since the age of three. It was at its worst at puberty. As a young child and before the psoriasis really took off, Rob was a keen swimmer and part of a local swimming team. He won a cup for swimming. But when the psoriasis took hold, Rob stopped swimming so regularly because of the problems of the communal changing rooms.

Rob has always worked hard at keeping his psoriasis under control, with varying degrees of success. He says that he considers the condition to be severe when it is on his face, scalp, arms, legs, chest and stomach. He finds it acceptable when it is just on his knee caps and the backs of his legs. He then feels relaxed enough to go out and socialise. Here is his story:

I was in hospital a lot when I was between the ages of 10 and 13. The psoriasis was on my face, scalp, knees, elbows, arms and legs. It was even in my nostrils. Sometimes when I would breathe out little flakes would come out like a snow storm. It was horrible, but that doesn't happen any more. I missed quite a lot of school during those years.

I would be more or less clear when I came out of hospital but it would start creeping back after about a week. The treatment at home was horrible. In the evening I would have the tar put on and then I'd be bandaged. On top of that I would wear really old pyjamas. My bed would be covered in bin liners with some old sheets on top and the pillow would have a bin liner wrapped around it with an old pillow case over it. Basically I was one great big bin liner.

There are no words to describe how much I hated it. My parents used to put the treatment on for me when I was younger and I used to get tense and up-tight and I really did not want to go to school in the morning or do anything. It made me feel grubby and dirty and I would smell a bit the next day. I'd put my track suit on and I could smell the tar on my track suit. The smell would come out in my sweat. But I never got any nasty comments.

I used to feel very resentful and wonder 'why me?'. It was like fighting a battle you weren't going to win.

I found it quite depressing at school. I couldn't relax or go into the shower with the other students because I'd feel they were looking at me even if they were not. I used to make sure that I was the last one to shower or I'd knock off 10 minutes early and be finished in the shower before the others arrived.

I enjoyed sport and I did play it but there were times when I was very reluctant to do so because of the state of my skin.

I've always enjoyed acting but I can remember once appearing in a school play as a maid and I had to wear a lot of heavy make-up. It made my skin blotchy and raw. I have to be very careful not to rub my face because if I do it will bring it up.

Sometimes when I wake up in the morning and the psoriasis is in a bad phase it makes me feel a bit down. I don't want to go out. It can be very depressing, especially if you are going out with someone. You want to look your best and although they accept you for who you are, you still feel bad about it. As much as you may try not to feel that way, you can't always shake yourself out of it,

I am forever putting moisturisers on myself and having moisturising baths, but the most beneficial treatment I have had is PUVA. I had to take the psoralen tablets two hours before the ultra-violet treatment and the tablets made me very drowsy. I kept wanting to nod off which made it difficult to work. And I had to wear shades all day. But I got a suntan and the psoriasis went. It came back after about a month.

In the summer my skin gets better. I try and sunbathe as much as I can, but I do it gradually. I remember one year when I was at college I was able to get home quite a lot and I would sunbathe in the garden most days for a few minutes. Within a couple of weeks my skin was smooth. You could see the outline of where the psoriasis had been, but my skin felt beautiful. My friends thought I'd been abroad. I tan easily and I'm convinced that if I lived in a hot climate I'd be clear of psoriasis.

I find the worst part of the condition is being self-conscious all the time and not being able to relax. That can get you down. I relish the day when I can go out and do a simple thing like wearing a T-shirt or rolling up my sleeves without worrying about the state of my skin.

I find shaving a nightmare. It's all right if I leave the hair to grow but as soon as I shave the psoriasis comes up a little bit. It means that when I shave I don't look my best. My girlfriend bought me an electric shaver for my birthday and I find that much better than razor blades.

But it doesn't get me down now as much as it used to when I was 18 or 19. I wasn't going steady with anyone then and I wondered if it was because of my skin. I think it was to do with the fear of rejection but that never really happened. I have a girlfriend and a job and now I look at it just as something that I've got. People seem to accept it. But I guess I just hope that some day soon it will go away . . .

11

ASPECTS OF LIVING

Psoriasis is a very individual illness. There are differences in how it appears on the skin and differences in the way the various treatments affect patients, as well as differences in each person's perception of it.

What also varies is in how people react to having psoriasis. Most people interviewed for this book have said that there are times when it is embarrassing and socially limiting. It is difficult to go out if your skin is looking awful or if you are tied down to a skin-care routine that is time consuming. The extent to which you can throw off feelings of diffidence and embarrassment differs from person to person. Some people can radiate a confidence that they may not really feel but it gets them out and about regardless of the vagaries of their skin, while others prefer to restrict themselves to the company of people with whom they feel safe. Most people seem to go to great lengths to keep their psoriasis hidden.

Patients also vary in how they handle other people's reaction to their skin. Some will say that they understand why, for instance, strangers do not want to occupy a swimming pool with them, while others will get angry at the ignorance and insensitivity displayed.

People without psoriasis vary enormously too. Some are naturally tactless and insensitive while many others are not. But the latter may initially need the person with psoriasis to meet them more than half way.

If you have never heard of psoriasis and haven't the faintest idea what it is, what would run through your mind when you were being introduced to someone who, for argument's sake, has a raw, flaky and uncomfortable-looking skin? Your first reaction may be that whatever it is, you don't want it. You may be irritated at being placed in a situation that may be potentially hazardous.

Our basic instinct is to protect ourselves. So in the same way as psoriasis patients may not want to go out when their skin is bad because they want to protect themselves from the remarks that may be made, non-sufferers, who are ignorant of the ailment may want to protect themselves from undesirable eventualities that they mistakenly believe may come their way. They may be bewildered or they may feel threatened and since you are the one with the information, you can do something about this.

If you can recognise the look that says: 'What is this? Will I catch it?' and answer the unasked question. 'I'm sorry about the state of my face/hands/scalp. It's psoriasis which is a heck of a nuisance for me but thank God it is in no way catching.' It not only informs nervous strangers but reassures them and puts them at their ease.

Of course it takes confidence and practice to be able to treat something that you feel vulnerable and sensitive about in such a casual way, but it is surprising how effective acknowledging a thing or situation can be in dispelling its power. Here's an example. You are at a party and a man supporting two very colourful black eyes is introduced to you. A variety of thoughts will go through your mind. You may think he looks a bit of a character or you may wonder if he is pugilistic by nature and want to remove yourself from his company. Whatever you may be thinking, the chances are that you will not be listening very attentively to what he is saying. Your mind will be somehow caught up with the state of his eyes.

However, were he to say something like: 'I feel such an idiot walking around with these two black eyes but I had a bump in the car and this is what I am left with.' The blackness of his eyes will suddenly become of so little interest that after a few minutes you may even forget to notice them.

Sometimes a condition like psoriasis can put sufferers on the defensive. It would not be remarkable for them to feel unjustly singled out for some very unfair treatment. A lot of patients have said that they wonder consistently 'Why me?' It can make you very resentful. You may feel that if someone is lucky enough not to have psoriasis, they should be thankful and therefore sensitive and caring to the people who do. After all, it is you who needs reassurance that you are wanted and valued despite the condition of your skin.

In theory this is true, but in practice it very rarely works that way. Managing the condition is not always just a question of attending to the skin, it can also include looking at what effect you, the person with psoriasis, has on the world around you in addition to examining what the world holds for you. And this may mean putting yourself in the place of uninformed non-sufferers and imagining how he or she feels in order to put them at their ease.

In this chapter we are looking at some of the different life-situations that most of us encounter with the object of discussing some practical ways of handling them. Please look at the section on teenagers on pages 110–11 for ideas on **clothes shopping** and **hairdressers**.

· *Family Life* ·

The same rules apply in family situations. We all need reassurance from time to time that we are important to our nearest and dearest. When we are ill this need to feel valued can become more obvious and, with a condition like psoriasis which can be chronic, the need to be reassured that we are loved, in spite of it all, can become quite acute and even unreasonable from time to time.

Inasmuch as psoriasis places a burden on the patient it can also be difficult for the patient's family. Even a very caring spouse may find it irritating to be constantly vacuuming dead skin and cleaning out the bathroom. They may love and support you but it doesn't mean that they won't get frustrated and upset by you if you forget to be considerate. Like anything else, consideration is a two-way street.

If you can, try to manage your psoriasis as much as possible yourself. Psychologically speaking, it is important to 'own it'. In other words, you say quite firmly to yourself that *you* have psoriasis. It does not belong to your wife, husband, partner, children, doctor or dermatologist. It's *yours*. It is part of you, albeit not the best part but, nonetheless, it belongs to *you*. This being the case, you have to take full responsibility for it. And this is not just in relation to your skin but to your immediate environment. You are in charge of keeping your skin moisturised and treated and you are in charge of seeking medical help if it starts to get beyond your control.

Equally, it is your responsibility to clear up after yourself. You may need to keep a small vacuum cleaner in the bedroom to use in the mornings. You may need to shake the sheets you have been sleeping on. It may be necessary to take a second look at the bath or shower after you have used it. Is it greasy or scaly? What about the basin? You may have to occupy the bathroom for a long time, so do so when it is not going to be in demand. Be aware that there may be ways in which you can help your family to cope with your psoriasis. This is not to say that the chores are not open to negotiation. You can share and you should accept all the support available, but it would be both caring and considerate to let your partner know that in the final analysis, as far as psoriasis is concerned, the buck stops with you.

From time to time most relationships go through bad patches which resolve themselves eventually. However, there are occasions when the stresses and strains of family life, added to another pressure like severe psoriasis, can be a little too much for couples to handle themselves.

If psoriasis is severe and if arthropathy (psoriatic arthritis) is involved, a couple's sex life can be affected.

If you are experiencing problems in your relationship, it may be worth considering seeing a couple counsellor. Relate, whose address appears in Useful Addresses, specialises in couple counselling. Many of the centres have a psychosexual therapist on their staff. The latter are trained Relate counsellors who specialise in helping couples with sexual problems.

· *Stress* ·

Where there is a predisposition to the condition, it is thought that stress may trigger an onset of psoriasis and if the condition already exists, stress may trigger a flare-up or make an on-going situation worse. No-one can get rid of stress in their lives, but what we can do is learn how to handle it – at least to some extent.

Our bodies are not really equipped to handle long periods of stress. Centuries ago when we were hunters the body was tuned to quick-action stress. When faced with a threatening situation we either stood our ground and fought or ran. This-fight-or-flight response has become part of our psychological and physical make-up.

When we prepare for action, the brain receives a warning signal. This triggers a chain reaction throughout the body. The adrenal glands secrete adrenaline and this mobilises the body's defences, preparing it to fight or run. The heart pumps more blood and more oxygen to the muscles. Blood vessels in the skin and stomach constrict to allow more blood to be diverted to the brain. The lungs bring in more oxygen. The body temperature rises and we start to sweat in order to cool down. Now another hormone, cortisol, is released by the adrenal glands. This is to gather energy from other parts of the body to stabilise the situation.

This was all very well for primitive man but it does not help us to cope with the kind of stress we are faced with today. The problem is that these days stress, pressure and anxiety can be with us day in, day out for months and years. So we have to find other ways of counteracting it. Sport is an excellent way of getting rid of the build up of adrenaline. But if that is not possible, try getting involved in a hobby, reading a good book, going for walks, doing aerobics, dancing, joining a gym or doing relaxation exercises, or meditating – just take time off to do the things that you enjoy.

· *Work* ·

There is no reason why a patient with psoriasis should not have a successful career in virtually any field of work. However, there are types of jobs that can cause problems because they may aggravate the condition. The jobs in this category include engineering, hairdressing, catering, domestic work and nursing. This is not to say that there are not many psoriasis sufferers happily and successfully employed in those careers, but there are circumstances in which problems can arise.

As was discussed in the previous chapter (see page 112), people with psoriasis on their hands may find that their condition gets worse when they are constantly exposed to water or chemicals. They may find it a barrier to getting jobs in the food industry. People with pustular psoriasis on the soles of the feet (see Chapters Two (page 19) and Six (pages 66–7)) may find that work which involves them being on their feet a lot of the time is more than they can easily cope with. Remember also that psoriatic skin damages more easily than normal skin and so manual work may not be suitable.

In some jobs it is possible to reduce the risks by wearing barrier creams and protective clothing. But this is not always the case. If you are having skin problems and you think they may be triggered by something at work, it is worth checking it out with a dermatologist to try to identify the culprit.

Patients with psoriatic arthropathy may not be able to manage physical work.

The police and the armed forces may not take on psoriasis sufferers because they feel that they may not be able to cope with all the aspects of the job.

It is very upsetting to be denied a job on medical grounds or to feel limited in the kinds of work you can do. But, at the end of the day, if the job you are doing is making your psoriasis worse or perpetuating it where it may otherwise remit, it may be worth looking for other work.

· *Holidays* ·

Holiday locations hold very few problems for people with psoriasis. Most sufferers prefer warm, sunny climates because sunlight can improve the condition. And if your psoriasis gets better in the sun, you can return from holiday relaxed, tanned and psoriasis-free. But you must be careful not to over-expose yourself to the sun because sunburn can make psoriasis worse (see Chapter Five, page 52).

If your psoriasis becomes worse in the sun, you obviously need to avoid those kinds of locations. If you cannot avoid warm, sunny places, use a sunscreen with a very high SPF factor, such as SPF 25 or 30.

Hotels can be a problem. Hotel staff can be very impatient when the floors are covered with scales and the sheets are soiled. Some psoriasis patients have been known to leave the hotel they are staying at ahead of schedule because of complaints or unkind comments from hotel staff.

You can get over this by taking with you a battery-held vacuum cleaner or a brush to pick up the scales, old sheets and pillow cases or a sleeping bag to place over the hotel's bedding and your own towels. Or you may just need to shake the sheets out in the bath in the morning if it is just dry scales that are involved.

Here are some other holiday tips:

- If you have a holiday planned and are on complicated or messy topical treatments, ask the doctor to give you something simpler to use while you are away.
- Take extra emollients and pack them in a hard plastic container to stop them from oozing out.
- If you can take more time with the moisturising, so much the better. Remember it will reduce, if not remove, the scaling.
- Don't forget the sunscreens.
- If you are self-catering, take extra bedding. Don't forget your washing up and cleaning gloves.
- Don't forget your medicines and take with you a list of your medication, your NHS number, and if you are travelling in Europe, the appropriate medical forms.
- In a hot climate, keep creams in the fridge. They will feel nice and cool when applied.
- If your skin is hot and itchy, fill a plastic bag with ice cubes and place next to the skin for instant relief.

· *Pregnancy* ·

The only reason to put off getting pregnant if you want to start a family is if you or your partner are on tablets that preclude this (see Chapter Four). Many women find that psoriasis gets better during pregnancy and some find that it stays the same. For a minority it can get worse. Some women find that shortly after the baby is born the psoriasis can deteriorate but this is temporary and eventually the condition settles down to how it was before.

· *Immunisation* ·

Having psoriasis is no reason to avoid immunisation. It is possible that the condition might flare up on the site of the injection just as it might through any other injury to the skin. Psoriasis that occurs in this way can be treated just the same as any other psoriatic patch. Immunisation prevents many fatal illnesses and it is almost always better to risk the possibility of triggering the psoriasis than getting the disease you are being immunised against. If you are unwell, particularly if you have a temperature, you may be advised to postpone the immunisation. This is true also, of course, if a child with psoriasis is due to be immunised. If you are unsure about your state of health, check with your doctor.

· *David* ·

David first had psoriasis in 1980. It came on soon after the birth of his first child and within months it spread all over his body. He was working as a bank manager at the time and had to put up with customers refusing to see him. In fact one called him a 'leper' and said that it wasn't right that the bank should allow someone like him to see customers. His colleagues, with whom he'd worked as a team for many years, were very supportive. Eventually David changed jobs but this was a personal preference and not to do with psoriasis. He is now a school bursar. He has two children. Here is his story.

My first child was born after my wife had had a series of miscarriages, a complicated pregnancy and an equally complicated birth. Miscarriages are very stressful and they affected my wife considerably. I tried to keep a stiff upper lip and I think I tended to push my own feelings to the back of my mind. I think the psoriasis came with the release of tension.

All through the pregnancy you are tense but the nearer it gets to the time when you lost your last baby the worse it gets. I can remember when my daughter was born. I held her within a few minutes and I was counting the number of fingers and toes to make sure she was all right. You think the miscarriages must have happened because something was wrong and this was a complicated pregnancy. So I feared some kind of defect. But my daughter was perfect.

I think that all the build up of emotion over the years which I wasn't able to show, came out at this time.

What actually happened was that I knocked my knee on an open drawer in a desk and a scab formed. My knee blew up and I had to have it drained. The doctor told me I had psoriasis on my knee and behind my ears. I didn't know what it was. I'd never heard of it before. Within about four months it engulfed my body. It looked like a sheet of wood-shavings. I was eventually admitted to hospital and it took them seven weeks to treat it.

I was very raw and inflamed so they began with emulsifying ointment for the first three or four days. Then they started building me up on coal tar which burnt me considerably. After a week they took me off coal tar and put me on dithranol. They started with a very low percentage and gradually built it up. After a couple of weeks that was burning me and it was nowhere near the strength that they were used to dealing with. By now I'd got a reputation!

They then tried Betnovate which was a little bit better and they put me on ultra-violet light which was quite successful. Since it wasn't such a mucky treatment it pleased me as well. I had four weeks of different coal tar type treatments and three weeks of ultra-violet light combined with Betnovate. The only tablets they gave me were sleeping tablets to make me relax and rest.

I was much better when I left hospital but within a couple of months it came back again and I went through a cycle where every couple of years I was admitted to hospital for long periods of treatment.

Subsequently, they prescribed Tigason and I have been on that ever since. I also have ultra-violet treatment and the combination of the two works well.

I was a bank manager when I first got psoriasis. It affected my work because customers would refuse to see me which made it difficult to do my job effectively. It caused problems in my married life because my wife didn't particularly like being covered in all the scales. She didn't want me near her so the physical relationship deteriorated. Although that didn't harm our relationship it did put pressure on it.

I joined the local branch of the psoriasis committee with another psoriasis patient who was on the ward with me. He has become a good friend of mine and now I am chairman of the committee and he is the secretary.

I came to terms with psoriasis very quickly and through it I have made some very good friends. I am one of those people who can actually say that, although I hate psoriasis, my life has benefited through it, because I have made a group of friends whom I otherwise would not have met. And that helps me to help other sufferers in their early stages by saying don't *let psoriasis hide you away. There are a lot of us out there who have got it and it can be a new social chapter for you.*

I have been through bad times with the amount of psoriasis I've had and the effect that it has had on me both at work and home. It has made me more tolerant of people who suffer in one way or another from an ailment. I think it's given me confidence to talk to people about personal things. People who come to our meetings will often say that things aren't so great at home. I don't get embarrassed. I explain my situation and I think it gives people the feeling that they are not alone.

On one occasion when my children were very little we went down to Bournemouth one weekend in the summer. It was hot and the beach was packed. There was nowhere for the children to dig sand castles. After a few minutes I started taking off my T-shirt and my skin was quite bad. My wife told me to put my vest on because people were looking. I didn't want to. I was feeling hot and I hoped that the sun would do something for my skin. Within 20 minutes the people around me had moved and my kids started digging sand castles. As more people came on the beach, they saw this bit of space and started unravelling their deck chairs, but as soon as they spotted me they went away.

My wife felt really embarrassed, but it gave the children the space they needed to build their sand castles. It took a lot of determination to just sit there. I think I try to disguise my basic lack of confidence by being over-confident at times. If someone else is suffering I will be the person to take the T-shirt off and say if I can do it, so can you. But it was a good four or five years after I first got psoriasis that I was able to do that.

What tends to happen now is that I have about two months remission and then the psoriasis starts to come back. For a month I have a lot of little patches in different parts of my body. Then the next month the psoriasis tends to take off. They put me on the PUVA and that takes about two months to work. I then have two months clear and it builds up again. I have about four months in a year clear. It's that kind of a cycle. I don't have long periods of remission but each time that I have the treatment it doesn't seem quite as bad as the last time so I feel I am winning.

As a governor of my children's school I appointed a deputy head. After he had started, I noticed that he had psoriasis all around his forehead. I told him that I had psoriasis too. He started coming to the meetings with me. He eventually married another teacher on the staff and I've got to know them both very well. They have recently had their first child and they have asked me to be her godfather. Through psoriasis we have a bond. And through psoriasis I have gained two very good friends and a goddaughter.

12

COMPLEMENTARY THERAPIES

Complementary therapies with their holistic approach now have a large following in Britain. Treating the whole person and not just the illness in isolation is a very attractive concept, as is the attempt made by these practitioners to effect a cure rather than just treat the symptoms.

Although there is very little evidence that any of these therapies will achieve the results that are sometimes claimed, many people do find some of the treatments therapeutic and there is no reason why you should not try any that appeal to you. Many of the therapies focus on reducing stress and promoting relaxation. Since stress can play a large role in perpetuating or aggravating psoriasis, learning to relax and unwind could certainly help to improve your skin condition.

Most complementary therapists will suggest that you continue with the treatment medically prescribed and it is important that you do this, particularly if your psoriasis is severe.

With so many different treatments on offer it is difficult to know which one to choose. Personal recommendation is a good starting point. If a friend tells you that his or her psoriasis has improved with a particular therapy, it may be worth a try.

As with other forms of treatment, it is essential to go to a qualified practitioner. There are no laws governing complementary medicine in Britain at present so anyone can set up in practice. However, therapists tend to belong to the appropriate professional body and these usually require that their members have passed examinations and reached the required standard. Contact the relevant professional body and ask them to recommend one in your area. Also remember that most complementary medicine is not available on the National Health, so it is well worth finding out the likely cost before embarking on any treatment.

This chapter describes a few of the many therapies that are currently available. For more information, contact the relevant professional body (for addresses, see 'Useful Addresses').

· *Acupuncture* ·

The word 'acupuncture' means 'needle piercing'. In China, where this treatment is practised widely it is called *Chen chiu*, which means 'needle moxa'. Moxa is a dried herb which is burned in small cones on the skin or on the handle of the needle to generate a gentle heat. This method is known as moxibustion. Both these methods can be used during acupuncture treatment.

Since the needles are so fine, there is no discomfort during the treatment but patients may feel a slight tingling. The needles may be left in for 20 minutes to half an hour or they may be withdrawn immediately. The moxa is burned on, or held near to the point and removed when the patient feels that it is becoming too hot. This process is repeated several times.

Children or adults who have a fear of needles are usually given another form of treatment. This includes massage and tapping or pressure with a rounded probe. Alternatively, they may receive electro-acupuncture and laser treatments in which the acupuncture points are stimulated either by a low frequency electrical current, applied direct with a probe, or with finely tuned laser beams. Gentle electrical stimuli may also be applied through the needles, giving a sensation of tingling or buzzing.

Acupuncture is part of a system of medicine that has been practised in China for several thousand years. Stimulation of acupuncture points induces the release by the brain of pain-relieving morphine-like substances known as endorphins. This may explain why acupuncture has been used as an alternative to anaesthetics in surgery.

Acupuncture is based on the principle that our health depends on the balanced functioning of the body's motivating energy. Known as *Chi,* this energy flows throughout the body but is concentrated in channels beneath the skin. These channels are called meridians and along them are the points by which the acupuncturist regulates the energy flow and bodily health.

The treatment aims to restore the harmony between the equal and opposite qualities of *chi*: the *yang* and the *yin*. *Yang* energy is aggressive, representing light, heat, dryness and contraction. *Yin* energy is receptive, representing tranquillity, darkness, coldness, moisture and swelling. A dominance of *yang* energy in the body is thought to be experienced in the form of acute pain, headache, inflammation, spasms and high blood pressure. An excess of *yin* can be felt as dull aches and pains, chilliness, fluid retention, discharges and fatigue.

Practitioners of acupuncture aim to discover the nature of the disharmony in the body. They do this by careful questioning and observation: they will examine the patient's tongue for its structure, colour and coating and feel the pulses for their quality and strength. Once the cause of the problem has been diagnosed, the acupuncturist will select the points and the appropriate method of treatment.

Some GPs practise acupuncture in their surgeries. Others will be able to recommend a qualified practitioner. If you don't want to go through your GP, you can find a qualified practitioner through the professional societies. Since needles are involved in the treatment, the big question mark is going to be hepatitis and AIDS. Members of these professional bodies have to use needle sterilization techniques approved by the Department of Health. These are considered to be effective against the hepatitis and AIDS viruses. Many practitioners use disposable needles.

· *Aromatherapy* ·

Practised widely in France, aromatherapy has been gaining a name for itself in Britain for the treatment of stress-related illnesses. Instead of drugs this therapy uses essential plant oils. An essential oil is what gives fragrance to a flower or herb. It is a liquid which is present in tiny droplets in the plants. Each essential oil has a number of different properties and it is the aromatherapist's job to evaluate which oil or mixture of oils will have a beneficial effect on a particular condition. For instance, some of the essential oils can have powerful antibiotic properties while others are effective with psychotherapeutic conditions. For psoriasis the essential oils of Bergamot and Lavender are often recommended. These two are often also used in preparations that are said to help you to sleep. Essential oils are used in a variety of different ways. They are often used as massage oils in which case the essential oil is blended into a 'carrier oil' which is usually an inexpensive oil that has no smell of its own. They are also incorporated into bath oils and can be used as compresses, inhalations and vaporizers.

When applied in the bath or directly on to the skin these oils are absorbed into the bloodstream and internalised in that way. However, it is said that there are some essential oils that have to be ingested to be effective.

With psoriasis there is always the possibility that you may get an adverse reaction to any particular oil so it is important to start very cautiously perhaps only trying one or two psoriasis-free areas in your body to see how it goes.

Although you can use aromatherapy on yourself, there are definite advantages in seeing a well-qualified aromatherapist who can mix a cocktail of oils that is specifically beneficial to you. Of course, seeing a therapist is much more expensive than the do-it-yourself treatment and aromatherapy needs to be maintained at home. Probably the best bet would be to go to a qualified aromatherapist for a thorough consultation. You should then be given the oils you need to use at home.

· *Homoeopathy* ·

Homoeopathy is the practice of treating like with like. The Greek word 'homoeo' means 'like'. Homoeopathy was invented in the 18th century by a doctor called Samuel Hahnemann who felt that human beings had a capacity for healing themselves and that traditional medicine had its limitations. Hahnemann believed that the symptoms of a disease were a reflection of a person's struggle to overcome harmful forces; the doctor's work should be to discover and, if possible, remove the cause of the problem and to stimulate the vital healing force of nature.

Dr. Hahnemann and his followers carried out experiments upon themselves. Over long periods they took small doses of known poisonous or medicinal substances, carefully noting the symptoms they produced (these experiments were called Provings). Patients suffering from similar symptoms were then treated with these substances with good results.

The next step was to establish the smallest effective dose in order to avoid side effects. To his amazement Hahnemann found that, using a special method of dilution, the more the similar remedy was diluted, the more active it became. He called this method potentisation. However, this paradox, that less of a substance could be more effective, was not at all acceptable to scientific thought at the time and Hahnemann and his followers were ridiculed.

These days homoeopathy is much more respected. The principles are still those established by Hahnemann. The patient is treated, not the disease. So the practitioner aims to get a picture of the patient as a whole. Along with the symptoms of the illness and the medical history, the homoeopathist will want to know about the patient's personality. He or she will ask questions about the person's temperament, likes and dislikes, particular aptitudes, as well as making a note of the person's appearance, skin colour, type and tone. It is said that all this helps to give the homoeopathist a whole picture of the patient and this is used to find the remedy that will suit him the best.

Remedies are prepared from animal, vegetable and mineral sources. They are diluted, using the process of potentisation that Hahnemann discovered, so that the patient receives an infinitesimal dose of the remedy which, paradoxically, achieves the maximum effect.

The British Homoeopathic Association can give you more information on this treatment and holds a register of homoeopathic doctors. Some GPs practise it in their surgeries and there are hospitals in various parts of the country that offer homoeopathy on the NHS.

· *Hypnotherapy* ·

In this treatment the aim is to shift the patient's attention from external to internal awareness. Much of the work goes on in the patient's subconscious mind. The hypnotherapist will want to try to assess, to some extent, the underlying cause of the problem. This may include finding out about the person's lifestyle, investigating causes of stress and other factors that may be triggering the condition or making it worse.

A medical history will be taken which will include finding out when the psoriasis started, what triggered it off and whether or not other members of the family have it. The hypnotherapist will also want to know whether the psoriasis is itchy or not because if it is, he or she may work on ways of controlling the itch.

Then the patient is put into a light trance state. This is a naturally occurring state, similar to day dreaming or the slowing down, drifting feeling before you drop off to sleep.

Hypnotherapists say that in the hypnotic state, people tend to be much more receptive to therapy in the form of suggestions and imagery. This is because the left side of the brain, which is in charge of analytical and logical thought, shuts off, allowing the therapist to communicate with the patient's subconscious mind without the blocks and defences that would usually exist. Most patients remember almost everything that has happened while in a trance state.

The hypnotherapist may now try to explore any possible underlying reasons which may be contributing to the condition. These could be feelings of stress and anxiety, poor self-image, lack of confidence and other negative thinking patterns.

Many therapists also employ visualisation techniques with their patients. For example, a patient may be asked to visualise in their mind that they are somewhere peaceful, such as lying on a boat and each gentle sway of the boat allows them to feel more relaxed. Or they may be asked to visualise a scene that has particularly restful connotations and imagine themselves there. People who are not good at seeing visual images in their minds can use their other senses to imagine being in a peaceful place like feeling the sun on their bodies, hearing the birds chirping, smelling sea breezes or evocative flowers, and so on.

This process can be emphasised by positive and soothing self-talk, such as the patient telling himself, 'I am feeling calm', 'I am in control', or, 'My body is feeling relaxed'.

The aim of the hypnotherapy is to make patients self-sufficient, so that they don't need to keep going for sessions of hypnosis. They are taught self-hypnosis. They are shown how to put in the appropriate imagery and how to phrase suggestions so that they can do it for themselves.

· *Meditation* ·

Many psoriasis patients interviewed for this book have said that they find being able to relax very helpful to their condition. Learning to meditate is for many people one of the best ways of learning to unwind and lower the stress factor. There are many different forms of meditation and which one you choose is entirely up to you. Yoga meditation is easily available and not at all difficult to learn. Most yoga teachers include it in their classes. Transcendental meditation, explained below, is easy to learn but quite expensive. Different forms of meditation suit different people and it can often be a case of trial and error before you find one that suits you.

At the very least, meditation should enable you to feel relaxed and still while you are meditating. If you meditate regularly you may find this feeling of inner quiet will stay with you, to a greater or lesser extent, in the course of a normal day.

· *Transcendental Meditation* ·

This technique, founded by Maharishi Mahesh Yogi, is not at all difficult to master. In a one-to-one session you are given a special sound or phrase called a *mantra*. You shut your eyes, quieten your mind and focus on the *mantra*. This helps to get rid of all the little thoughts that race across your mind. Eventually, you let go of the *mantra* and achieve a deep sense of stillness and inner quiet. The meditating sessions last between 15 and 20 minutes, but the feeling of peace stays with you, to some extent, throughout the day. As you become a regular meditator – and you are supposed to do it twice a day – this inner peaceful feeling is constantly replenished and emphasised. It is as simple as that.

For a stress-related condition like psoriasis, transcendental meditation can be very helpful. Research has led to the discovery that, while sleep triggers the body's restorative powers, the deeper state of mental relaxation achieved during meditation allows this repair work and recuperation to be carried out more efficiently.

Learning the technique doesn't come cheap but it is a one-off payment that lasts for life (subsequent check-ups, if you need them, are free). It is a seven-stage course which you can learn in about a week.

· *The Radiance Technique*® ·

The Radiance Technique® is also known as The Authentic Reiki. Practitioners of this therapy observe that too much emphasis is placed on outside healing and the possibility that people have an essential part to play in promoting their own health, or recovery from illness, is largely ignored. So The Radiance Technique®, also referred to as TRT, aims to enable people to access their own universal energy and in so doing promote healing along with a feeling of well being. There is also an accent on promoting personal and spiritual growth.

The Radiance Technique was apparently understood in ancient Tibet thousands of years ago. The belief was that people could learn to access cosmic transcendental energy through the power of touch. In by-gone years there were known keys that activated this natural energy and this information was passed from teacher to student by word of mouth.

Eventually this knowledge found its way into other parts of the Far East including China and Japan where it was translated into symbols and buried in ancient and obscure languages. In the mid-19th century Dr. Mikao Usui, a Japanese scholar who was able to read Sanskrit (an ancient Indian language), discovered in some ancient Sanskrit texts the symbols appertaining to this knowledge. Today, a formula, based on these series of symbols, apparently starts a process by which students of TRT tap into the natural energy of the universe and bring about a change in their physical, spiritual and emotional circumstances.

The therapy is based on a (w)holistic view of the human being which is the basis of most complementary therapies. Therapists here spell the word with a 'w'. They say that people need to develop a perspective in their daily lives of seeing themselves in terms of organic wholeness. This necessitates being aware of their own internal being as well as the external one. It means that they should become aware of themselves, physically, mentally, emotionally and spiritually and understand that it is a combination of all these things that makes them who they are.

The theory is that since all these aspects of your person combine to make you yourself, you cannot adequately treat an illness by just attending to one bit of the package that is you – in other words the physical part. To bring about healing you have to attend to the wholeness of yourself. Equally, if you want to live life to the full and make the most of the energy-force around you and within you, you have first to shift to this wholistic view which will enable you to reach a consciousness that will vitalise your entire being.

Practitioners say that you cannot learn this therapy from a book. You have to attend classes given by teachers who have been properly trained and attuned to the process. Students can learn individually or attend classes or seminars. In her book, *The 'Reiki' Factor in The Radiance Technique*, Dr. Barbara Ray, the foremost international authority on the technique, explains the procedure: 'TRT accesses natural, whole energy which can in one aspect of its use be systematically directed as a physical therapy. In brief, TRT hands-on sessions begin at the top of the head and in four steps cover the eyes, the sinus tracts, the brain, the pituitary and pineal glands, the throat, and the thyroid gland'. Students are taught how to place their hands on those parts of the body in order to activate energy.

In the first part of this process, the anatomy from the neck upwards is covered. The next part, which again involves placing your hands in strategic positions, involves the heart, lungs, liver, stomach, intestines and so on and finally you cover the rest of your body including the lower back, kidney, spinal cord and adrenal glands.

There is apparently a direct relationship between some of our glands and the natural energy centres in our body and our emotional and spiritual well being.

The Radiance Technique can be practised alongside any other therapy – medical or complementary – and by any age group. It is not a religion. Students can learn the process at varying degrees of expertise from one to seven. The first seminar, which is a 12-hour course, gives you what is called by TRT therapists 'The First Degree'.

In The Second Degree, students who want to go further into TRT begin a discovery process with cosmic symbols. They learn to 'direct energy outside time and space' for absent healing. They can then use TRT for family and friends at a distance when they may not be able to give them a hands-on session.

Ingrid St. Clare is a TRT teacher who has completed training to The Sixth Degree. At the age of 14 she was covered in psoriasis. It was all over her body and on her hairline and she was acutely embarrassed by it. 'I didn't go swimming and wore clothes that covered me because if I didn't people would comment,' she says. She treated it unsuccessfully with steroid creams.

Thirteen years ago when she was in her mid-thirties she decided to learn The Radiance Technique. This was not in an attempt to clear her psoriasis but because she was interested in spiritual growth. She says that after she completed The First Degree her skin started to improve but it was a very gradual process, with it getting better at times and worse at others over the next three years.

'I had been living in America for a while and when I came back to England my psoriasis got worse. I thought it was due to the extra stress and I spent extra time doing TRT on myself,' she explains. 'One way of healing is that it all comes out and that could have been what was happening because after that last flare up it hasn't come back. And that was 10 years ago.' Occasionally, an injury like an insect bite may trigger a psoriatic patch but it is a small one and does not cause Ingrid any problems.

The First Degree is a 12-hour course. After this you become self-sufficient in applying the technique on yourself and you don't have to take it any further to benefit. In this first seminar you receive what the therapists call an 'attunement' process. Apparently the teacher tunes you into the universal energy which enables you to access it.

You also learn how to use the 'hands on technique' (as described above) which you are instructed to do every day. In addition to reducing stress and promoting relaxation, the 'hands on' exercise apparently balances the different systems in our bodies, including the natural energy centres, and this helps us to maintain and improve our health. Learning meditation is also part of this first seminar.

Training is usually in small groups and the hours of the seminars are fitted in to the students' requirements. Three sessions of four hours each is usual.

The Reiki Factor in The Radiance Technique and other books on TRT are published by Radiance Associates. If you are interested in learning this technique you should contact the Radiance Technique Association for Great Britain for a fully accredited teacher.

· *Reflexology* ·

As with the other complementary therapies, Reflexology aims to help the whole body to function more efficiently. Applying pressure to minute points on the soles of the feet is thought to relieve stress-related illnesses by releasing endorphins, morphine-like chemicals in the brain. Each zone of the foot corresponds to a different part of the body (limbs and internal organs).

The principle is that if the patient feels pain when the therapist is massaging a certain zone in the foot, it may reveal problems in the correlating part of the body. It is apparently a very relaxing and soothing treatment.

· *Shiatsu* ·

This therapy promotes relaxation and relief from stress. *Shiatsu* is a Japanese word which means 'finger pressure'. The theory behind *Shiatsu* is very similar to that of acupuncture in that the person stays healthy when the flow of energy circulates unimpeded around the body. Pressure is applied to various parts of the body which correspond with the meridians used in acupuncture. The *Shiatsu* practitioner can apply pressure on the meridians by using his/her thumbs and fingers or elbows and sometimes even knees and feet. This apparently stimulates circulation and the flow of lymphatic fluid. It apparently works on the autonomic nervous system, helping to release toxins and tensions from the muscles and, it is claimed, it can also stimulate the hormonal system.

Treatment usually starts with a diagnostic session when the practitioner will examine the person's face which, they say, gives a great deal of information about their state of health. Blemishes, lines and colour changes all have a significance to the *Shiatsu* practitioner. Touch is extensively used as a diagnostic tool and the timbre of the voice is also thought to be an indication of a person's health. 'Hara' diagnosis is sometimes used, which involves palpitating the abdomen to find out the energetic quality and balance of the various internal organs. *Shiatsu* practitioners say that they can also diagnose from the pulse.

Shiatsu is complementary to orthodox medicine and practitioners will often give advice on diet and exercise. The length, frequency and total number of sessions varies according to individual need.

· *Spiritual Healing* ·

Spiritual healing is said to be the channelling of healing energies through the healer to the patient. Its purpose is to re-energise and relax the patient and allow the latter's own natural resources to deal with the illness or injury. By directing energy, usually through the hands, the healer aims to supplement the depleted energy of the patient, deal with stress at whatever level it exists and release the body's own recuperative abilities.

Healing can be given for any illness, stress or injury, and apparently people receiving it can experience sensations of deep relaxation or energy. Some experience a pins-and-needles sensation, feel hot or cold, and some feel pain coming to the surface and dispersing which is said to be an indication that the treatment is working.

In their leaflet on spiritual healing, The National Federation of Spiritual Healers say: 'The power of nature to enable us to help ourselves, recognised for thousands of years, has been overshadowed in modern times by the growing emphasis on technology. It is this power which spiritual healers seek to tap, addressing illness and injury at its source and aiding recovery at all levels of the patient's being.'

The rationale is that spiritual healing penetrates the person's being at a deep level where many illnesses have their origin. When the cause of the illness is discovered and removed, symptoms disappear.

However, the NFSH advise their patients to contact their doctors about conditions which may require medical attention and that healing is not a substitute or alternative but can work very well as a complement to other forms of treatment.

The National Federation of Spiritual Healers represents more than 7,000 members, bound by a strict code of conduct, who work individually and in centres throughout the country. It is a registered charity and operates through regional committees. It is not associated with any religion or -ology.

The fee for spiritual healing can vary. Some healers do not charge at all while for others it is their sole source of income.

· *Yoga* ·

Yoga is a system of mental, physical and spiritual development which originated in India three thousand years ago. The word 'yoga' comes from an Indian word meaning 'to unite' and is said to be a means of restoring a healthier balance to body and mind, enabling the person to cope better with the stresses and strains of everyday living.

In a yoga class you will probably start by learning a series of stretching exercises that enable the body to become more supple. These postures are not just physical exercises but a way of gaining greater control over body function. Yoga 'asanas' (postures) gently stretch and contract every muscle in the body. Joints are encouraged to move more freely resulting in improved posture and, it is said, greater stamina and vitality.

If your psoriasis is severe you may find these exercises are impossible to do without splitting the skin. So you may have to give it a miss. Similarly, if you have arthropathy (psoriatic arthritis), you should not embark upon the physical exercises in yoga without discussing it first with your doctor or rheumatologist.

The emphasis in yoga is very much on individual development. The fact that someone else in the class is exceptionally supple is not considered to be of relevance to you. Some yoga teachers ask their class to keep their eyes closed while doing the asanas so as to increase concentration and bring home the non-competitive nature of the exercise.

You may also learn breathing techniques. Yogis have used breath-control techniques for centuries as a means of improving health and vitality. They say that these techniques, practised in the right way under the guidance of a good teacher, can be a means of improving respiration generally.

The classes almost invariably finish with a period of relaxation, when students are taught how to direct the mind to different parts of the body and instruct them to relax. This is followed by a period of deep relaxation.

Meditation is an important adjunct of yoga teaching. Different methods are used to quieten or concentrate the mind so as to achieve an inner silence.

If you are interested in taking up yoga, make sure the teacher is qualified. Most of the postures take a certain amount of learning and it is important to get them right. Group classes are not usually expensive and they can be quite sociable. The British Wheel of Yoga is a well established organisation with qualified teachers who run classes throughout the country.

13

THE PSORIASIS ASSOCIATION

The Psoriasis Association was started in 1968 by a dermatologist at Northampton General Hospital and his psoriatic patients. Dr. Dick Coles had spent many years running group therapy sessions for his patients. People with psoriasis would meet in Dr. Coles' house and talk in a relaxed and informal way about the problems of having psoriasis.

It was quite an insightful and innovative thing for Dr. Coles to instigate as, until then, treatment had focused very much on the physical aspects of the illness with the psychological and emotional issues being side-lined.

In an article in an early edition of the journal of The Psoriasis Association, Dr. Coles describes those early gatherings. 'Our group meetings involve psoriasis sufferers who have attended our out-patient clinic and received an invitation to join a few others one evening in a discussion of common problems. We begin by listening to a short talk about psoriasis together with a few slides, all conveniently available on a simple audio-visual TV set. This outlines in straightforward terms the nature, probable causes and treatment of psoriasis and introduces a few ideas on the problems of coping with it.

'The talk thaws the ice by giving the group members an opening for questions and ideas of their own. A free discussion follows in which the sufferers themselves express their own views and offer experience and advice to one another. Helping oneself and helping one another are therefore just as important as learning facts about psoriasis.'

Dr. Coles goes on to explain that although the group therapy sessions could not cure the condition, nor directly control the symptoms, it aided improvement by getting rid of the anxieties experienced by sufferers and helped them to develop a 'sensible approach towards the condition and its treatment'. He says: 'Psoriasis can become less of a struggle dominating one's life and more of a limited problem affecting only one part of the body'.

From these beginnings the idea of setting up a formal self-help group that would enable psoriasis sufferers all over Britain to meet, exchange ideas and support was mooted.

Eventually, with very little money, the Association was founded. It was registered as a charity and it ran solely on private donations.

Today The Psoriasis Association has a membership of more than 12,000 people and has become an important self-help organisation providing support and mutual aid for sufferers. The Association is managed by an elected council of voluntary members supported by a small number of full-time employees. The Association is advised by a Medical and Research Committee and each year supports more and more research projects into the causes, treatment and cure of the condition.

The Psoriasis Association has become the main source of information on all aspects of psoriasis and has forged close links with similar organisations throughout the world. One of its main aims is to raise standards of patient care through its contacts with the medical profession, the social services, government departments and other organisations.

Membership is open to anyone. Every member receives the national journal *Psoriasis* three times a year. This includes articles by sufferers as well as medical experts on all aspects of the condition.

A number of local groups affiliated to the national body meet regularly to provide points of social contact and information as well as to raise funds for research and educational projects. Members can participate voluntarily in the activities of these groups.

Linda Henley, the current National Secretary, joined the Psoriasis Association in 1973. She had always been aware of the condition since several members of her family suffer from it. She became National Secretary in 1978. She says that one of the most significant changes she has noticed since she first joined the Association has been the shift in doctors' and dermatologists' attitudes towards the condition.

'In the early days a self-help group, particularly for skin sufferers, was unheard of and they didn't know quite how to take us,' she says. 'They didn't know if we were going to be a threat, gang up on them or cause problems by grumbling about everything.

'But there were also some very good people in the medical profession who helped us over the years and now the situation has changed. They understand that we are here to help patients in a very different way.'

Since its inception The Psoriasis Association has given over a million pounds to psoriatic research, including various projects looking into the efficacy of different psoriatic treatments like PUVA baths, for instance.

Doctors are beginning to identify the genes that predispose people to psoriasis. A recent project has involved taking blood samples from patients where there is a strong family connection with psoriasis. Doctors have been extracting the DNA from these blood samples in order to do molecular genetic studies.

Dr. Jonathan Barker, a consultant dermatologist at the St. John's Institute of Dermatology, who is heading the London part of the study, says that once doctors are able to discover the genes that cause psoriasis they will be able to develop much more specific therapies to treat it. 'Potentially, you may be able to cure the illness. You will certainly be able to counsel people. Some patients with psoriasis want to know what likelihood there is of their children developing the condition. This information should potentially become available.'

· *In The Family* ·

Muriel first had psoriasis when she was 12 years old. She is now 82. She recalls that it first appeared after she had visited a relative in Stockport. During the visit she had met an old man with a glass eye. He had frightened her by staring at her hard and she had found it very unnerving. Soon after that the psoriasis came on. However, the first appearance of psoriasis was also coincidental with the birth of her sister Audrey.

Muriel comes from a family of five – four girls and one boy. Her brother never had psoriasis, but three of the girls did. The fourth girl died when she was 32, so it is possible that psoriasis may have made an appearance later on had she lived. Neither of Muriel's parents had it.

Muriel's psoriasis has been with her in varying degrees of severity ever since it first appeared in 1925. She has had it on different parts of her body at different times with the elbows and legs being the most common sites. But there have been times when it has covered very large areas of her body. She remembers the old days when psoriasis would rear its head 'just when a dance was on'. She says: 'That was the worst part. I'd have to wear long-sleeved dresses which the seamstress would have to make up very quickly.'

Muriel has never been to see a specialist about her psoriasis. It was always treated by her GP. She was given coal-tar treatments to do at home which she remembers as being both messy and smelly. Her daughter, Belinda, however, recalls the tar with some affection. 'I can remember as a child having to rub my mother's legs with the tar. Even to this day I find the smell of it very evocative,' she says. Belinda suffers from a mild form of scalp psoriasis as does her son.

These days Muriel treats her condition only with emollient (E45) which she finds 'marvellous'. Muriel is convinced that, for her, stress plays a large part in how severe the psoriasis is at any given time.

Psoriasis came on much later in life for Muriel's next sister. Beryl was in her twenties when it first appeared and she was due to go with her husband to live in India. Although Beryl coped with the condition very well in India, once she returned to England the psoriasis deteriorated and she had it fairly severely right up until the time that she died.

The youngest of the three girls, Audrey, first got psoriasis when she was five, but for her it has always been fairly mild. Very fair-skinned, with gingery hair (unlike her two sisters), Audrey's skin is sun-sensitive and even as a child she would have to be careful to keep out of the sun or cover up.

Psoriasis has reached the third generation of the family with some of the children and grandchildren of the three women suffering from it, but none severely.

The Psoriasis Association is open from 9am to 5pm, Monday to Friday. The address is on page 154.

A–Z of Psoriasis

Acitretin

This is a retinoid treatment for psoriasis (see Retinoids). It is the generic name for Neotigason.

Alcohol

Alcohol can sometimes aggravate psoriasis, but it can usually be tolerated if taken in moderation. However, if the patient is on the drug Methotrexate, alcohol should be avoided as it could increase the risk of liver damage.

Calcipotriol

This is a relatively new topical treatment for the treatment of moderate to mild psoriasis and is a derivative of vitamin D. It is sold under the brand name of Dovonex. Calcipotriol is thought to work by reducing the excessive reproduction of skin cells that cause the thickening and scaling and produce the psoriatic patches. It is particularly good for treating chronic plaque psoriasis and it doesn't stain or smell. But calcipotriol can irritate the skin and produce a rash on the face even if it is not being applied there. An excessive use of calcipotriol can raise the level of calcium in your body which can cause problems.

Cigarette smoking

Smoking has been linked with pustular psoriasis.

Common plaque psoriasis

Also known as chronic plaque psoriasis, this is the most common form of psoriasis and usually appears on the scalp, lower back, outsides of the elbows and knees, and the shoulders. Each psoriatic patch looks like a series of little discs or plaques that have superimposed themselves on to the body. The plaque-like shapes are peculiar to this form of the condition and are what gives it its name. Common or chronic plaque psoriasis is an adult condition, seldom seen in children. Treatment includes ointments and creams, tablets and ultra-violet. Many patients find that natural sunlight can help their skin, providing they do not overdo it and allow their skin to burn.

Corticosteroids

These are artificially produced hormones which are sometimes used to treat psoriasis, particularly in the form of ointments or creams. They do not cure the condition but they reduce inflammation and itchiness. Unfortunately, once you stop using them the psoriasis usually returns. This is known as the 'rebound effect'. There are side effects if steroids are used constantly.

Cortisone creams and ointments

These preparations include a small percentage of steroids (see corticosteroids) in a carrier ointment or cream.

Curatoderm

This is the brand name for Tacalcitol.

Cyclosporin

This is a drug treatment for patients with severe psoriasis. Used mainly for transplant patients as it suppresses the rejection of transplanted organs, it can also be very effective in treating psoriasis.

Cyclosporin is an immunosuppressive drug which works by dampening down strong allergic and immune reactions. It also has anti-inflammatory properties. But it can have some very serious side-effects and is therefore treated with caution.

Day-care clinics

These clinics enable patients who would normally have been admitted to hospital to have such treatments as tar baths, tar applications and dithranol on a day-care basis in the hospital's dermatology unit. This service is invaluable to patients who need the treatment but cannot afford to spend time as an in-patient. It also solves the hospital's problem of providing beds. Treatments given on a day-care basis are quite varied and they do not have to be complex to qualify for the day-care programme.

Disability living allowance

This is a tax-free social security benefit for people under 65 years of age who have an illness or a disability and need help with getting around or help with personal care or both. If you are over 65 you may be able to receive an Attendance Allowance for help with personal care. Although you are unlikely to need a medical examination, you do have to prove special needs to qualify. There are two components to DLA – care and mobility.

If you can only walk a short distance before you feel severe discomfort, you may qualify for DLA on the mobility component.

You can get DLA for mobility for children who are five or over, but they must need a lot more help than children of the same age who do not have a disability.

You could qualify for the care component if you need help with washing, dressing, using the toilet or if you need someone to keep an eye on you. You can claim this benefit for children and babies of any age but they must need a lot more help than children of the same age who do not have a disability.

For both the mobility and care component you must be likely to need help from the date of your claim for six months or more.

If you want to know more, ring the Benefit Enquiry Line Freephone 0800 882 200.

Disability working allowance

This provides for people over 16 who are working or starting work but whose income is limited because they have an illness or disability. You need to be working for 16 hours or more a week in paid employment. You may be eligible if you already receive DLA or have been getting one of the following benefits in the last eight weeks: Invalidity Benefit, Severe Disablement Allowance or a disability premium with Income Support, Housing Benefit which includes a disability premium or council tax benefit which includes a disability premium. You can apply if you have less than £16,000 in savings but any savings between £3,000 and £16,000 will affect the amount of DWA you receive. You can pick up a claim pack to apply for this allowance from a post office or Social Security office. You can get more information from Freephone 0800 882 200.

Please note that the details on both the Disability Working Allowance and Disability Living Allowance change from time to time so it is advisable to check with the telephone number above.

Dithranol

This is a man-made chemical and one of the most successful treatments for psoriasis. It is particularly effective for common or chronic plaque psoriasis. It can be a little messy to use and can cause burning so treatment needs to be monitored.

Dovonex

This is the brand name for calcipotriol, a topical treatment for psoriasis.

Emollients

These are simple moisturisers which you apply to the skin to keep it from drying. Emollients do not heal psoriasis but they can help to reduce itchiness and prevent the skin from cracking. Used regularly, they also greatly reduce scaling. Generally, these moisturisers do not have any side effects but some people may find that certain brands irritate the skin, for instance, if the moisturiser contains perfume and the patient is allergic to perfume. If a particular moisturiser produces any kind of irritation or inflammation, change to another brand. Moisturising the skin regularly is the first-line treatment for psoriasis.

Erythrodermic psoriasis

This is a rare but serious condition in which the rash is spread over large sections of the body. The skin is very inflamed which affects its ability to function properly. It does not retain fluid as normal which results in the patient feeling constantly thirsty and being dehydrated. It also impairs the skin's performance in maintaining the body's temperature control. This condition needs expert medical management. When so much of the body is affected it is unlikely that creams and ointments will be enough to bring the condition under control so the patient will almost certainly require drug treatment.

Facial psoriasis

Psoriasis that appears on the face can be very distressing because it is so visible. Keeping the face well moisturised is an important part of the treatment but your doctor can also prescribe preparations that do not show up on the skin but can help to clear the condition.

Women with facial psoriasis may find wearing a thick foundation useful for hiding the lesions and beauty therapists can be very helpful. It might be best to book a private consultation in a salon rather than going to a beauty counter in a department store.

Men may find shaving a problem as it can aggravate psoriasis. Dry shaving, with an electric razor, is usually best and applying a moisturiser after you have shaved will keep the skin supple. If you are worried about looking greasy, gently blot the face after you have moisturised with a thin piece of tissue and the rest will evaporate very quickly.

Feet

Psoriasis that appears on the soles of the feet is known as pustular or palmar planter psoriasis. It can be very troublesome. The doctor can prescribe topical treatment to help. Resting your feet as much as possible is important. Walk around at home bare-foot so that the air can get to your feet. At other times wear cotton socks and leather shoes that allow the feet to breathe.

Flexural psoriasis

This type of psoriasis only appears in the folds or creases in the body. The most common sites are the armpits, the skin underneath the breasts and the groin. There is very little scaling although the patches are inflamed and can feel very sore. The condition very rarely appears on its own and is much more likely to accompany common or chronic plaque psoriasis. Making sure that the folds of the skin are gently patted dry after washing can, sometimes, stop the condition from developing, and if it is already there, make sure that the skin folds are kept dry. People who are overweight are more susceptible to this condition.

Generalised pustular psoriasis

This is a rare but serious form of psoriasis in which pustules are spread over large sections of the body. Patients suffer high temperature often accompanied by pains in the joints. The sufferer is ill and requires professional medical management and is likely to be treated in hospital.

Guttate psoriasis

This form of psoriasis is most commonly experienced by children. It usually appears suddenly, often following a bacterial throat infection. The skin condition usually appears about two to three weeks after the infection and spreads quite quickly all over the body apart from the palms of the hands and the soles of the feet. The patches are red and scaly and an attack rarely lasts more than a few weeks. Guttate psoriasis is quite easily treated, usually with ointments and creams, and 50% of sufferers who receive effective treatment never seem to have another attack. With other patients, common or chronic plaque psoriasis can ensue.

Hands

Psoriasis that appears on the backs of the hands is usually common or chronic plaque psoriasis but when it is on the palms of the hands, it is pustular psoriasis, also known as palmar planter psoriasis. Keeping your hands protected is an essential part of self-help treatment. Wear protective gloves when doing housework or DIY. Cutting or bruising your skin can trigger psoriasis which is why it is so important to look after this often over-worked but very vulnerable part of your body.

Heliotherapy

This is the name for sunlight therapy.

Itching

Over 50 percent of psoriasis sufferers experience itchiness, particularly if the condition appears in the scalp. Psoriasis comes from the Greek word 'Psora' which means 'itch'. Itching is an integral part of psoriasis.

Dry skin that cracks is more itchy than moisturised skin. Over-heated rooms are a great promoter of itchiness. Keep the room cooler rather than hotter but not too cold. Low humidity and bad ventilation can also make you itch. So keep the windows open.

Some people become itchy if they use soap and very warm baths can also make you itchy.

Some people find that woollen clothes worn next to the skin can make them itch. Cotton is better. Also look out for scratchy seams, labels and materials in the clothes you wear. Tight clothing can make you hot and itchy. Wear loose-fitting garments that give your skin a chance to breathe.

Methotrexate

This is a powerful anti-cancer drug which is sometimes used to treat generalized pustular psoriasis, generalised psoriasis and psoriatic arthritis. Taken over a long period of time it can damage the liver and it can also have an effect on the production of red and white blood cells. Patients on this treatment need to have regular blood tests. They are also strongly advised to avoid alcohol.

Nails

Psoriasis that appears on the nails of the fingers or toes can be difficult to treat because topical preparations are messy to apply and they don't stay on easily. Fingernails tend to be pitted and the nail can become discoloured or it can separate slightly from the nail bed. Should the nail go a greeny-black colour, seek medical attention because there may be an infection present. Nail varnish can hide the blemishes.

Neotigason

This is a retinoid treatment for psoriasis (see Retinoids, pages 47–8). It is the brand name for acitretin.

NSAIDs

Non-steroidal anti-inflammatory drugs are commonly used to treat psoriatic arthritis. They relieve stiffness, pain and inflammation of the bones and joints.

Prescription charges

If you are spending a lot of money on prescriptions, think about getting an NHS Certificate of Prepayment of Charges. This way you pay a set amount, either annually or quarterly, and all your prescriptions are covered for that period, whether you have one or 101 prescriptions. Ask your chemist for the relevant form.

Psoriasis

Psoriasis is a skin complaint which occurs when new cells are produced much more quickly than normal before the old skin cells have been shed. This results in the new cells accumulating on the surface of the skin, producing patches of thick, inflamed skin covered by scales. Psoriasis can sometimes be accompanied by a special form of arthritis.

Psoriasis can appear for the first time at any age and it is thought that sufferers inherit a predisposition to it through family genetics. Once started, it can recur throughout life. It is often triggered by emotional stress or trauma or sometimes by an illness. Although psoriasis cannot be cured, there are many treatments that can heal the psoriatic patches and help to keep the condition under control.

Psoriasis is **not catching**. Nor is it a form of skin cancer. It is an autoimmune disease.

The Psoriasis Association

This is a well established self-help group for psoriasis patients and their families. It was started in 1968 by a dermatologist, Dr. Dick Coles, and his patients. Its aims are to raise the standards of patient care and provide up-to-date information on psoriasis to psoriatic patients and the general public. Through its journal the Association keeps members in touch with the latest research and medications available. Local groups, affiliated to the national body, allow people with psoriasis to get in touch with each other for mutual support.

Psoriatic arthritis

Symptoms of this are very similar to the more usual form of arthritis with the joints becoming swollen, tender and very painful. The most common sites for this complaint are the finger joints, toe joints, feet, part of the jaw and spine. It is very important to get this condition diagnosed as early as possible because without proper treatment it can deteriorate. Treatments available include ointments and creams, drug therapy, physiotherapy and ultra-violet light therapy. With good medical care psoriatic arthritis is unlikely to result in permanent disability.

PUVA

This treatment combines the use of the UVA band of ultra-violet light and chemicals extracted from plants known as psoralens. Psoralens can be taken by mouth in tablet form or applied to the skin as either paint/emulsion or added to water (Bath PUVA). Ultra-violet light is always given prior to the application of topical treatments. PUVA treatment is useful for common or chronic plaque psoriasis, guttate psoriasis and pustular psoriasis. It is always carried out in hospitals and is carefully monitored. PUVA treatment can increase the risk of contracting skin cancer.

PUVA baths

This is essentially PUVA treatment but instead of having to swallow a psoralen tablet, patients are asked to have a bath in which a psoralen solution has been added prior to having the sunlight therapy.

Research

Doctors believe that they may have identified the genes that predispose people to psoriasis. This could have several ramifications. Patients with the condition may be able to assess the likelihood of passing on psoriasis to their children. Perhaps more importantly, it may lead to the development of more targeted medication, produced especially for psoriasis, that can control or even cure the condition.

Retinoids

Related to vitamin A, these are a systemic treatment for psoriasis. They work by reducing the production of keratin which is the protein that forms on the outer layer of the skin and gives it the thick, horny appearance. The retinoid tablet used for psoriasis is acitretin which is the generic name for Neotigason.

Salicylic acid

Salicylic acid is a topical treatment which works by removing the layers of dead skin cells. It is particularly useful for treating crusts and thick scale in scalp psoriasis. It is often used as a compound preparation.

Scalp psoriasis

This is one of the most common forms of the condition. Lesions can appear in the visible areas of the scalp with the forehead along the hairline being a common site. The nape of the neck, temple, around the ears and the hair parting are also likely places for the condition to appear. Scalp psoriasis is very uncomfortable and can also be extremely itchy. Scratching and picking makes the psoriatic patches sore and they can start to bleed. Scalp psoriasis is *not* caused by poor hygiene or hair care and it does not permanently affect hair growth. Hair that may fall out during a flare-up of psoriasis grows back once the condition has abated. There is a wide variety of shampoos and hair lotions to treat the condition and many of these are available without a prescription.

Skin

This is the largest organ in the body and its main functions are to contain and protect the internal organs and to stop the body fluids from oozing out. It also plays an important part in temperature control. When the skin function is damaged, as it is in severe forms of psoriasis, several things can happen. The temperature control mechanism can be impaired which means you can feel very hot or very cold in situations where this would not normally occur.

In acting as a barrier, the skin protects the internal organs from infection. When there are many psoriatic lesions in the body, the skin is much more open in those areas and there is a much greater risk of infection being introduced into the body through the damaged skin. You may feel unusually thirsty when the condition is severe and this can be caused through damaged skin letting the water out of your body much more easily. It can also make your skin feel very dry. Drinking non-alcoholic drinks can counteract this as can regularly moisturising the skin.

Stress

Although there is no evidence that stress can cause psoriasis, there is a lot of evidence that if you already have psoriasis stress can make it worse. For many people the flare-up can occur during stressful times, but others cope very well during periods of stress and experience a deterioration in their skin when the stress is over and everything has settled down.

Fun is a good antidote to stress. If you can make a point of doing something you really enjoy at least every week, if not every day, you will have something to look forward to which can help to counteract feelings of tension and stress.

Sulphasalazine

The brand name of this drug is Salazopyrin. It is usually prescribed for the treatment of bowel disease, but it is also sometimes used, in much smaller doses, to treat psoriatic arthritis as well as rheumatoid arthritis.

Sunbathing

Many people with psoriasis find that sunlight has a beneficial effect on their condition. Treated with caution, sunbathing can speed up the healing process. However, sunburn can make psoriasis worse. In the first few days of sunlight, expose your skin very gradually to the sun, increasing it bit by bit every day. But take care not to overdo it. If you notice any signs of sunburn, moisturise your skin and cover up immediately.

There are some medicines that make your skin extra sensitive to sunlight. Some antihistamines can do this, as can drugs taken for arthritis and other conditions. If you are on any medication, check with your doctor that it does not interact with sunlight.

Some patients with psoriasis are not helped by sunlight.

Sun protection factor

Included in a sunscreen, this provides your skin with protection from the sun's rays. The higher the SPF, the greater the protection. People with pale skin should use a sunscreen with an SPF of 15 or more. People with darker skins may be able to get away with a SPF 10 sunscreen but if in doubt it is better to go for one with a high SPF than risk burning with a lower one. Some patients with fair skins have found that using a sunscreen with a very high sun protection factor, SPF 30 for instance, can minimise problems.

Systemic medicines

These are drugs that you take into the system, usually in the form of tablets or injections.

Tacalcitol

Sold under the brand name of Curatoderm, this new topical treatment works by slowing down the production of new cells. It is a derivative of vitamin D. Tacalcitol needs to be used sparingly on the site of the psoriatic lesions only. It is applied once a day, preferably at night and can be used on the face.

Tar

Tar is a traditional treatment for psoriasis that has been successful for many patients for many years. Its drawback is that it is smelly and troublesome to use but it does heal the patches.

Topical treatment

This consists of creams and ointments that you apply directly to the skin and it is the most widely used form of treatment for psoriasis. Topical treatments can be simple moisturisers which you use every day to keep your skin soft and supple even if the psoriasis is clear. Other topical treatments are the tar, dithranol, salicylic acid, steroid creams and compound formulations that you use to bring an attack of psoriasis under control.

Triggers

There are several things that may trigger psoriasis in susceptible people. Stress is thought to be one. This is not to say that stress causes psoriasis but if you already have the condition or have a predisposition to it, stress – either emotional or physical – can trigger a flare-up. It is virtually impossible to rule out emotional stress in one's life but you can take steps to counter-balance it by relaxing, taking regular exercise and making sure that you take time off to enjoy yourself. Physical stress is caused by working long hours without enough rest and nourishment.

Some medicines can trigger psoriasis and these include beta-blockers, Non-Steroid Anti-inflammatory Drugs (NSAIDs) and Lithium.

Bacterial throat infections are a trigger and skin injury can often set off the condition, sometimes in an area of the body where it hasn't occurred before. If you cut or bump your skin it can set off psoriasis as can insect bites, skin infection and sunburn.

Alcohol can make the condition worse for some sufferers. Being overweight increases the body folds and renders you more prone to flexural psoriasis.

UVB

Many psoriasis patients receive UVB treatment. Ultra-violet B is the shorter wavelength of light that produces the sunburn. UVB treatment is given in a similar way to PUVA but with UVB no psoralens are taken either in systemic or tablet form.

Weather

Excessive heat can aggravate psoriasis and many sufferers may find an electric fan a big help in the summer. Cold winds can be very drying to the skin and make the psoriasis worse. Keeping well wrapped up if you are going out for walks on a cold, windy day is important. You may also find that you need to use more moisturisers during the winter months.

USEFUL ADDRESSES

Please note that if you require information to be sent to you, most of the organisations listed request that you send them a stamped addressed envelope.

Arthritis Care
18 Stephenson Way
London NW1 2HD
0171 916 1500

The Arthritis and Rheumatism
Council
Copeman House
St. Mary's Court
St. Mary's Gate
Chesterfield
Derbyshire S41 7TD
01246 558033

Benefit Inquiry Line
0800 882 200

British Acupuncture Association
34 Alderney Street
London SW1
0171 834 1012/6229

British Association for Behavioural
Psychotherapy
c/o Harrow Psychological Health
Services
Northwick Park Hospital
Watford Road
Harrow
Middlesex HA1 3UJ
0181 869 2326

British Association for Counselling
(BAC)
1 Regent Place
Rugby
Warwickshire CV21 2PJ
01788 578328

British Association for the Person-
Centred Approach
BM BAPCA
London WC1N 3XX
(Has a list of qualified members)

British Association of
Psychotherapists
37 Mapesbury Road
London NW2 4HJ
0181 452 9823

British Homoeopathic Association
27A Devonshire Street
London W1N 1RJ
0171 935 2163

British School of Reflexology
92 Sheering Road
Old Harlow
Essex CM17 0JW
01279 429060

British Society for Medical and
Dental Hypnosis
01709 554558

The British Wheel of Yoga
1 Hamilton Place
Boston Road
Sleaford
Lincs NG34 7ES
01529 306851

Cotton On
Monmouth Place
Bath BA1 2NP
01225 461155

Disabled Living Foundation
380-384 Harrow Road
London W9 2HU
0171 289 6111

Institute of Complementary Medicine
PO Box 194
London SE16 1QZ
0171 237 5165

Institute of Psychoanalysis
Mansfield House
63 New Cavendish Street
London W1M 7RD
0171 580 4952

International Psoriasis Treatment
Centre
Ein Bokek
Dead Sea
Israel 00972 7 584484
FAX: 00972 7 584390

International Society of Professional
Aromatherapists
ISPA House
82 Ashby Road
Hinkley
Leicestershire LE10 1SN
01455 637987

National Federation of Spiritual
Healers
Old Manor Farm Studio
Church Street
Sunbury-on-Thames
Middlesex TW16 6RG
01932 783164

National Register of Hypnotherapists
and Psychotherapists
12 Cross Street
Nelson
Lancs BB9 7EN
01282 699378

Psoriatic Arthropathy Alliance
P.O. Box 111
St. Albans
Herts AL2 3JQ
01923 672837

The Psoriasis Association
Milton House
7 Milton Street
Northampton NN2 7JG
01604 711129
Fax: 01604 792894

The Radiance Technique
9 Finedon Hall
Finedon
Northants NN9 5NL
01933 681900
or Susan Howell
01273 422437

Regional Health Information
Service
0800 665544

Relate
Herbert Gray College
Little Church Street
Rugby
Warwickshire CV21 3AP
01788 573241

St. John's Institute of Dermatology
St. Thomas's Hospital
Lambeth Palace Road
London SE1 7EH
(Please note that you have to be
referred to St. John's by your GP. The
hospital cannot act as a helpline or an
information source.)

Shiatsu Society
5 Foxcote
Wokingham
Berks RG11 3PG
01734 730836

Tisserand Association of Holistic
Aromatherapists
65 Church Road
Hove
East Sussex BN3 2BD
01273 772479

Transcendental Meditation
Freepost
London SW1P 4YY
0800 269 303 (Freephone)

Karen Michaels
VIP Health Holidays
42 North Audley Street
London W1A 4PY
0181 952 2059

Westminster Pastoral Foundation
23 Kensington Square
London W8 5HN
0171 937 6956

ACKNOWLEDGEMENTS

I should like to thank Linda Henley, National Secretary of The Psoriasis Association for the help she gave me in writing this book, and for her unfailing enthusiasm. I should also very much like to thank Dr. Jonathan Barker, Consultant Dermatologist and Senior Lecturer at The St. John's Institute of Dermatology, for reading the manuscript and advising on medical accuracy. Many thanks to Lynette Stone of The St. John's Institute of Dermatology for the help and advice on hospital procedure and my thanks also go to Dr. Roman Gumon of The International Psoriasis Treatment Centre in Israel for his help on Dead Sea treatment. Finally I should very much like to thank all the psoriasis patients who talked to me about their condition, many of whose personal accounts appear in this book.

INDEX